THE SUBFERTILITY

VIRGINIA IRONSIDE is a journalist who writes a regular advice column for *Today* and another column for *The Independent*. Formerly agony aunt at *Woman* magazine and the *Sunday Mirror*, she is well known for her honest and sympathetic approach. She is the author of 15 books, both fiction and non-fiction. She has some personal experience of subfertility and is a patron of CHILD. She lives in North London and has one son.

SARAH BIGGS began her career as a diagnostic radiographer, then in the pharmaceutical industry before working as an information officer in a specialist fertility clinic.

As a result of her own experiences of infertility she wrote *The Infertility Handbook* (Fertility Services Management, 1989) and went on to become Vice Chairman of CHILD, the national infertility support group. She served on the Kings Fund Committee, set up to consider the counselling needs of assisted conception patients, and currently serves on the Inspectorate of the Human Fertilisation and Embryology Authority. She is married with an adopted son.

Overcoming Common Problems Series

For a full list of titles please contact
Sheldon Press, Marylebone Road, London NW1 4DU

Overcoming Common Problems Series

Fight Your Phobia and Win
DAVID LEWIS

Getting Along with People
DIANNE DOUBTFIRE

Getting Married
JOANNA MOORHEAD

Getting the Best for Your Bad Back
DR ANTHONY CAMPBELL

Goodbye Backache
DR DAVID IMRIE WITH COLLEEN
DIMSON

Heart Attacks – Prevent and Survive
DR TOM SMITH

Helping Children Cope with Divorce
ROSEMARY WELLS

Helping Children Cope with Grief
ROSEMARY WELLS

Helping Children Cope with Stress
URSULA MARKHAM

Hold Your Head Up High
DR PAUL HAUCK

How to Be Your Own Best Friend
DR PAUL HAUCK

How to Cope with Splitting Up
VERA PEIFFER

How to Cope with Stress
DR PETER TYRER

**How to Cope with Tinnitus and Hearing
Loss**
DR ROBERT YOUNGSON

How to Do What You Want to Do
DR PAUL HAUCK

How to Improve Your Confidence
DR KENNETH HAMBLY

How to Interview and Be Interviewed
MICHELE BROWN AND GYLES
BRANDRETH

How to Love and Be Loved
DR PAUL HAUCK

How to Negotiate Successfully
PATRICK FORSYTH

How to Pass Your Driving Test
DONALD RIDLAND

How to Solve Your Problems
BRENDA ROGERS

How to Spot Your Child's Potential
CECILE DROUIN AND ALAIN DUBOS

How to Stand up for Yourself
DR PAUL HAUCK

**How to Start a Conversation and Make
Friends**
DON GABOR

How to Stop Smoking
GEORGE TARGET

How to Stop Worrying
DR FRANK TALLIS

How to Survive Your Teenagers
SHEILA DAINOW

How to Untangle Your Emotional Knots
DR WINDY DRYDEN AND JACK
GORDON

Hysterectomy
SUZIE HAYMAN

Is HRT Right for You?
DR ANNE MACGREGOR

The Incredible Sulk
DR WINDY DRYDEN

The Irritable Bowel Diet Book
ROSEMARY NICOL

The Irritable Bowel Stress Book
ROSEMARY NICOL

Jealousy
DR PAUL HAUCK

Learning from Experience
A woman's guide to getting
older without panic
PATRICIA O'BRIEN

Learning to Live with Multiple Sclerosis
DR ROBERT POVEY, ROBIN DOWIE
AND GILLIAN PRETT

Living Through Personal Crisis
ANN KAISER STEARNS

Living with Grief
DR TONY LAKE

Overcoming Common Problems Series

Living with High Blood Pressure
DR TOM SMITH

Loneliness
DR TONY LAKE

Making Marriage Work
DR PAUL HAUCK

Making the Most of Loving
GILL COX AND SHEILA DAINOW

Making the Most of Yourself
GILL COX AND SHEILA DAINOW

Making Time Work for You
An inner guide to time management
MAREK GITLIN

Managing Two Careers
PATRICIA O'BRIEN

Meeting People is Fun
DR PHYLLIS SHAW

Menopause
RAEWYN MACKENZIE

The Nervous Person's Companion
DR KENNETH HAMBLY

Overcoming Fears and Phobias
DR TONY WHITEHEAD

Overcoming Shyness
A woman's guide
DIANNE DOUBTFIRE

Overcoming Stress
DR VERNON COLEMAN

Overcoming Tension
DR KENNETH HAMBLY

Overcoming Your Nerves
DR TONY LAKE

The Parkinson's Disease Handbook
DR RICHARD GODWIN-AUSTEN

Say When!
Everything a woman needs to know about
alcohol and drinking problems
ROSEMARY KENT

Self-defence for Everyday
Practical safety for women and men
PADDY O'BRIEN

Slay Your Own Dragons
How women can overcome
self-sabotage in love and work
NANCY GOOD

Sleep Like a Dream – The Drug-Free Way
ROSEMARY NICOL

A Special Child in the Family
Living with your sick or disabled child
DIANA KIMPTON

Stop Smoking
BEN WICKS

Talking About Anorexia
How to cope with life without starving
MAROUSHKA MONRO

Talking About Miscarriage
SARAH MURPHY

Think Your Way to Happiness
DR WINDY DRYDEN AND JACK
GORDON

Trying to Have a Baby?
Overcoming infertility and child loss
MAGGIE JONES

**Understanding Obsessions and
Compulsions**
A self-help manual
DR FRANK TALLIS

Understanding Your Personality
Myers-Briggs and More
PATRICIA HEDGES

Vasectomy and Sterilization
Making the right decision
SUZIE HAYMAN

A Weight Off Your Mind
How to stop worrying about your body
size
SUE DYSON

Why Be Afraid?
DR PAUL HAUCK

You and Your Varicose Veins
DR PATRICIA GILBERT

You Want Me to Do *What*?
A guide to persuasive communication
PATRICK FORSYTH

Overcoming Common Problems

THE SUBFERTILITY
HANDBOOK

Virginia Ironside
and Sarah Biggs

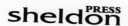

First published in Great Britain in 1995 by
Sheldon Press, SPCK, Marylebone Road, London NW1 4DU

The source of the information given in all the figures and graphs is derived from
research conducted at The University of Bristol, Department of Obstetrics and
Gynaecology, St Michaels Hospital, Bristol. Some of the data is reproduced from
'A Population study of causes, treatment, and outcome of infertility', a clinical
paper published in *The British Medical Journal*, 1985, and is redrawn with the kind
permission of Professor M. G. R. Hull and *The British Medical Journal*.

British Library Cataloguing-in-Publication Data
A catalogue record for this book is available from the British Library

ISBN 0–85969–707–X

Photoset by Deltatype Ltd, Ellesmere Port, Cheshire
Printed in Great Britain by Biddles Ltd, Guildford and King's Lynn

Contents

Acknowledgements

Virginia Ironside would like to thank CHILD for their help.

Sarah Biggs would like to thank Professor M. G. R. Hull and Liz Corrigan of the University of Bristol Department of Obstetrics and Gynaecology for their enormous help, and also Ben Plumley of the Human Fertilisation and Embryology Authority.

To Jack and John
SB

Introduction

This book is designed to help those who find they are unable to start a family when they are ready to. The stresses and emotions of subfertility are explored in detail, along with information about diagnosis and treatment.

The text is addressed to you as a couple, but certain sections refer to each partner specifically. To simplify the text, where the section is headed with ♀, the information that follows is addressed directly to the female partner; where the section is headed ♂ the information is addressed directly to the male partner. This is not to ignore the many single women who have concerns about their fertility and who seek treatment to help them have a child in the absence of a partner. The information in this book provides information useful to couples and individuals equally.

This book deals with what is commonly referred to as 'infertility', but a more appropriate term for those who experience some delay in starting a family would be 'subfertility', which implies a reduction in fertility rather than a complete inability to achieve conception.

We hope you will find the book helpful and we wish you every success and happiness, whether you achieve your desire to have children or not.

1
So you want to have a baby

It all seemed so easy, didn't it? You just decided to get pregnant, stopped taking the Pill or threw away your cap or your condoms, and waited.

And then you waited. And waited, And waited a bit more. And then you worried. And then you told yourself not to be so silly and waited.

And then you panicked. *Maybe having a baby wasn't going to be so easy after all.*

To find that, for you, getting pregnant isn't easy, upturns everything you have been told from your mother's knee. However liberal and unsexist your upbringing, if you're a girl you will have almost certainly played with dolls, mothering them from an early age as practice for what seemed like an inevitable future. And then, after puberty, the issue that's preoccupied most of our sexual and love lives has been that of trying desperately *not* to become pregnant. Parents have worried, teachers at school have warned, books have been thrust into your hands telling you all about contraception, magazines have underlined that it is possible for women to become pregnant at any time in their cycle at all, agony aunts have cautioned that the withdrawal method is no good because of the risk of minute leakages during intercourse . . . 'getting pregnant' has been a kind of mythical bogeyman that can happen to anyone if they aren't permanently on the look-out.

There are hundreds of family planning clinics around, and magazines are filled with advertisements for abortion clinics. *Not* getting pregnant is big business, and sometimes one could be forgiven for wondering how on earth the human race manages to reproduce, so much money, research, time and energy is devoted to stemming the flow of babies.

But not for you. You seem to be swimming against the tide. You *can't* get pregnant, and you feel absolutely awful.

You and your partner will never, it seems, become what society thinks of as a 'real family'. Society feels uncomfortable with the idea of subfertility or infertility. It sees a normal family as a father,

3

mother, and two children. People around you feel happier if they can pigeonhole you as mother *or* career woman. If you have been married or in a stable relationship for some years, friends and strangers alike tend to enquire about your plans for a family, and, no matter how strong your defences and how cogent your reply, the pain caused is considerable. 'What I wanted was not so much to be Mr and Mrs,' said one woman, 'It was to become part of a new family, a family of my own. And whatever people may say, Mr and Mrs simply isn't a family. It's a couple.'

Then, the prospect of subfertility or infertility rocks the very foundations of our own sexuality. 'There is something about the idea of a "barren woman" that conjures up such a horrible image', wrote one woman who had problems becoming pregnant. 'I always imagine her, withered and thin, like one of those miserable creatures in the Bible. Sometimes it almost seems like a sin, being barren'.

These feelings of being unfeminine or unmasculine, mere dry sexual 'nothings', are just some of the painful spin-offs arising from subfertility and infertility. Men suffer, but many of them appear to take subfertility more in their stride than women. It could be because they are naturally more emotionally repressed or because they have been brought up to channel most of their creativity into work, but, for some men, children might well be the be-all but not the end-all as well. (But, for men from cultures in which it is extremely important to a male ego to have a child, failure to produce can be a dreadful blow to masculine pride. After all, if the culture says that to have a daughter rather than a son is pretty bad, imagine what that culture says when you can't produce anything at all.)

In Western society, however equal the sexes have become, it is the mother who bears the child and, if research into parental behaviour is correct, still change 99 per cent of the nappies and spend by far the most time with a baby and small child. And therefore most, if not all, women, feel that their femininity is undermined when they are beset with fertility problems. Their longing to mother, their driving maternal instinct, is every bit a physical and emotional craving as that suffered by a heroin addict desperate for a fix. One would-be mother wrote to *CHILDCHAT*, the magazine for CHILD, the self-help group for people with fertility problems (for their address, see page 144) and put it like this:

I feel I have so much love to give and nowhere to channel it. It is entirely a different love that I have for my partner . . . I feel that part of me is dying inside and withering away. I feel that most women (and some men) with children view me as incomplete or not a real woman beause I have failed to join 'the club' and conform to society's expectations which are instilled and conditioned into us in our formative years, etc. – girls play with dolls, boys with cars, girls take parentcraft classes, boys do wood or metal work and suchlike.

Therefore it is not easy to cancel out your 'training for life' (or for your hormones, for that matter). Even in the human biology class when reproduction is explained, everything is taken for granted. 'This is what you do and then you get a baby.' In our teens, contraception is rammed down our throats to avoid unwanted pregnancies, therefore males and females are left in no doubt that they are highly fertile beings, who are all capable of reproduction. Nothing prepares you for discovering the opposite, does it?

Then there are the overwhelming feelings of powerlessness over a body that simply doesn't seem to function effectively, a powerlessness that soon seems to seep into other areas of your life as well. You feel completely at sea.

What will your future bring? When a woman is not at work she may find that she has more time to brood about the absence of a child in her home. This is also true where both partners are not working. One of the few advantages of unemployment is that parents have more time to spend with their children and so, in the absence of absorbing hobbies, childless couples may feel an even greater sense of loss.

But if you're in work, other problems arise. Should you continue struggling up the career ladder or would it be more sensible to give up work, if that is possible, and take things easy at home, trying to 'relax'? How on earth can you keep your job if you need time off for tests, without letting on that you're trying to get pregnant? After all, if everyone knows you're trying, they may pass you over for promotion, assuming you'll be successful eventually. But if you're not successful, then you would have liked to have tried to further yourself in your career. Most women usually do their best to keep quiet at work about their attempts to get pregnant, tying themselves into knots of excuses to get away from work for all kinds of appointments that, because of the ways our bodies work, simply cannot be changed. If you have been taking drugs to stimulate ovulation and need to go for an ovary scan, there is no way you can change your appointment to a week later. If you can confide in an immediate boss, so much the better, but you may have to weigh up the balances of whether you feel able to do this or whether confiding about your attempts at pregnancy might put your job under threat.

Job problems, yes, and holiday problems as well. First, if you are having expensive treatments, can you afford holidays? 'Altogether we spent about £6000 on GIFT, IVF and AIH,' wrote one woman who had successfully conceived, 'but that's nothing compared with what some people spend. I was lucky. When Bradley was born and I held him for the first time I felt like a proper woman and wife at last. Giving birth you're fulfilled. It's something to be proud of.'

In her case her money was well-spent, but all too often money can appear to go down the drain on unsuccessful fertility treatment. Where do your priorities lie? There follow all kinds of worries about finance. Should a holiday be taken when the money might be spent on fertility treatment? Would the relaxation gained by going on holiday be worth it? And if you are going in for fertility treatment, can you even spare the time to get away? Would you actually relax on holiday if you were worried anyway, and so on.

How can you make any plans at all? What will your future be? What may have seemed a neat package, indeed what may have seemed the only reason for getting married in some cases, has suddenly become uncertain. You may have decided to get pregnant, give up your job, and have a baby. But what now? Should you let out the spare room that you had ear-marked for the baby? What will happen in the future? Will it just be the two of you, for ever, ending up in an old people's home alone, with no one to visit? What is the point, you may ask, of living, if there is no one to care for, no one to be a physical expression of you and your partner's love for each other, no one to carry on your genes? If, at the very bottom, we are here to further the race, what is the point of life if we can't?

These feelings of powerlessness and complete lack of control over the future inevitably make us feel angry. And angry, usually, about everything. Couples may feel furious with their stupid doctor, who never told them that after a year of unsuccessful trying, they could be referred to a fertility clinic, enraged when a member of their family becomes pregnant, livid to read about couples abusing their children, hopping mad with each other, perhaps blaming each other for their problems, full of resentment and rage against friends who make insensitive remarks like; 'You don't want to leave it too late, do you?', and tremendous anger, ultimately, with themselves. The frustration of not becoming pregnant can lead to physical problems, like acute anxiety; and then that anxiety may be blamed, probably wrongly, for contributing to the fertility problem. 'Relax!' you may keep yelling at yourself, in a voice full of tension, your whole body wound up like a spring. You may get mysterious aches and pains, and headaches, and look every symptom up in a medical book hoping against hope that backache, tearfulness, cramps, and insomnia are signs of pregnancy. But they're not. They're the physical symptoms of pain and loss.

Often friends will be muttering that the more relaxed you are, the more likely you are to become pregnant. There is absolutely no evidence to show this, but because of a desire to feel in control, we often prefer to blame ourselves for our bodies' physical failings, even though it may be very unfair, just to give us the illusion that we have some power over the situation. Then we wonder if we shouldn't take tranquillizers to calm us down. Then we worry if tranquillizers will affect conception. And so on, tossing and turning throughout the night.

As fertility counsellor Jennifer Hunt says:

'It is quite common for couples to be so shocked at the initial diagnosis that they are numbed and unable to comprehend the facts laid before them. Carefully prepared life-plans are suddenly jeopardised by the spectre of infertility, their senses of reality and normality recede, and they may talk of "living in a nightmare". The stuff of nightmares is fear, confusion, feelings of being powerless and out of control, threat of violence or violation and all too often an overpowering sense of loss.'

One of the things we may mourn is the loss of the opportunity to pass on things to our children that we were given in our own family, or things that we were not given but wish we had been. Much of the satisfaction of childrearing is in trying to put right one's own childhood by getting it right for one's child. Giving a child a happy and secure home can almost compensate for not having a happy and secure home oneself. You want to put right that which was wrong in your own past.

Because of the social taboo about talking about being subfertile, there is a strong tendency to keep the information to oneself, too. This can make one much more isolated. And any subfertile couple often learns to keep quiet simply because of the reactions they've had from friends when they have made the mistake of opening up about their problem. 'If you go on holiday you'll get pregnant', they'll say, glibly and unthinkingly. Or 'Why don't you adopt? You'll get pregnant then.' In other words, they may just churn out stupid old wives' tales that do nothing to make couples with fertility problems any happier. You well know that these recommendations are based on anecdotal, not scientific, evidence. From your first consultation on, you'll know more about fertility than any of your childbearing friends. You will learn to be experts in the field, but friends continue with a barrage of well-meaning but, ultimately, cruelly uneducated advice: 'You must relax . . .', 'You should make love more often . . . less often', 'They say that there's a hill in Glastonbury that if you walk around. . .', 'My friend got pregnant out of the blue when she . . .', and so on.

Then there are those who say, 'You're lucky not to have kids –mine are little monsters, bless them.' How dearly you would love to have children to call 'monsters'! And how angry you feel with your friends who dare be so blithely secure about their fertility that they can speak so frivolously. To you this kind of remark is as offensive as a rich man who pushes away food he's too full to consume, in front of a starving child.

Then there are the remarks like, 'Lucky you, without kids you'll be able to do exactly what you want!' But what you *want* of course, is to have a baby, so that's a stupid thing to say, like saying to a man in a wheelchair, 'Lucky you, you can just doss around all day.'

Or, worse, there are the kinds of jovial comments made by insensitive men to subfertile fathers in pubs, along the lines of 'I see you're not firing any bullets yet!'

You can sympathize with the sad feelings experienced by the woman quoted below who, like so many with fertility problems, instinctively feared confiding in anyone else, at least not to anyone who couldn't sympathize from personal experience:

My problem is that I find it extremely difficult to discuss my infertility with friends and family. I very much want to talk about this to my family and gain another ear to listen to my hurt and sadness, but I feel as though they may not understand what I am feeling inside, hence I put on a brave face and continue with my life as normal (without the baby I do want). I have a son from a previous relationship who is now 11 years old and myself and my husband love him very much, but my need for more children causes me hidden grief and guilt for feeling such a way.

8

It really is important to be able to find people to talk to who are in the same ghastly situation as you. It is a rare friend, unless they have experienced the pangs and pains of subfertility themselves, who can really comfort you, however sympathetic they may be in other ways, but if you can find such a friend, then 'coming out' about your fertility problems can bring unexpected rewards. Experts have estimated that as many as one in six couples will experience some difficulty in achieving a pregnancy, which means that someone you know, maybe even someone you know well, *does* know exactly how you feel and can help you share the experience. Talking with other men and women who have experienced the same feelings, the same pain, will help you begin to come to terms with your own situation and so help you overcome it.

Along with the feelings of isolation and anger, other common feelings are disbelief, denial, guilt, and despair. Researchers conducting a study into the effects of subfertility found that half of all couples involved in the study felt that their subfertility was the most upsetting experience of their lives. Another study of subfertile patients found that 40 per cent of women and 16 per cent of men demonstrated a clinically significant level of depression.

But worst, by far, is the terrible feeling of loss and bereavement. Many people talk about their feelings of bereavement as being particularly difficult because it is a sense of loss about something that does not exist. Jennifer Hunt, though, disagrees: 'Many of my clients have a real sense of what a baby would be like. They know full well what they are missing. They can imagine their baby as if it is real.'

But what is difficult is that this feeling of mourning is for something that is not tangible, either physically or socially. There are no funeral services for the subfertile. No one writes letters of condolence. Only the most sensitive of friends will ever even acknowledge that the hope of having a child is remote. On the whole they will jolly you up with tales of surprise pregnancies: 'I know someone who was kissed on the head by the Dalai Lama, and she became pregnant, you never know!' 'I know this person who got pregnant at 48! It's never too late!' But sometimes it *is* too late, or it is pretty likely to be impossible. And the feelings of longing, the desperate hope, combined with the feeling of guilt and misery that the chances are so very slim, can result in dreadful unhappiness.

The following letters are poignant reminders of how desperate those who grieve, and those who long for the feeling of a baby in their arms, can feel. And knowing of others' pain might, I hope, make you feel less alone.

My husband and I have been married for four years. We've had lots of good times but the last year has been hell, for one reason only. We would love to have a baby and I am undergoing fertility treatment at the moment. We both realize that this may take up to two years. At the moment, however, I hate going anywhere, to see friends, to parties, even to weddings, because everyone is always talking about babies.

All our friends have kids and I just feel so left out of conversations and general chit-chat. I feel so desperate that I don't even want to pick up a baby now because I feel so jealous.

My husband tries to be sympathetic and understanding but he always seems to say the wrong thing at the wrong time. We always seem to argue about the smallest things, yet we love each other so much. If anyone asks, I always say we wouldn't even consider having a family yet. I could not bear the thought of everyone knowing that I couldn't have kids and everyone feeling so sorry for me. Because of this I feel like I am under so much pressure all the time, that there are times that I just feel that I cannot go on with life because without a baby our lives are so empty and incomplete. It makes it so much harder because we both love each other so much and we want to share our love with our own child. I just feel that this problem is going to cause the break-up of our marriage, which is the last thing that we want. But I just do not know where to go from here. I feel so desperate, and emotionally unstable. Please help.

A letter to God

Dear God
Please tell me that I'm not going to feel like this for ever. Please make the pain and hurt go away. I feel as though I'm in a living hell from which there is no escape. Each morning I wake and promise myself that today I will be positive, cheerful and nice to everybody. But it's there all the time like a big shadow cast over your whole life. The thoughts are there through each waking hour and at night the nightmares take over. Please God, tell me that I'm not going mad. Please help me learn to like myself. Please let me have the child I long for. Please God.

Now you know that you're not alone, that the feelings you're having are perfectly natural, perhaps you want to take more positive steps.

You may be subfertile at the moment, but is your problem one that can be solved? What are the treatments available? How do you get them? And how far do you want to travel along what could be a very long road indeed?

Read on . . .

2

The facts of fertility

♀ ♂ *Statistics*

It is difficult to establish accurately the number of couples who are unable to start a family when they choose to. Estimates vary between as many as one couple in every six to one in ten. These estimates are unlikely to include many of the considerable number of couples who suffer secondary infertility, that is, couples who already have one or more children by a current or previous partner.

Of those couples for whom a reason for their failure to conceive can be identified, it is estimated that approximately one-third can be attributed to the male partner, one-third to the female partner and one-third to a combination of both partners.

There has been surprisingly little data collected on a national scale about fertility, conception rates, and the incidence of subfertility in the population as a whole. One report, dating back to 1956, revealed that 90 per cent of all fertile couples will conceive within a year of trying, and that after 2 years of trying, up to 95 per cent will be successful.

In contrast, the general population, which includes subfertile couples, can expect that only around 85 per cent will conceive within the first year of trying, rising to 90 per cent after two years.

It is not thought that subfertility as a whole is on the increase, but the slight decrease in the number of couples who could expect to conceive within a year could be attributed to some of the social changes that have occurred since 1956. Today, many women work for a number of years before contemplating a family, and, as fertility is known to diminish with age, this may increase the length of time taken to achieve a pregnancy.

There has been some publicity, mainly in Europe and the United States, suggesting that there is a global decrease in sperm counts, giving rise to increased subfertility. It is hard to assess this as it is based on the results of semen analyses performed in the late 1940s and early 1950s and, subsequently, in the 1970s on a substantial group of men, which have been compared with analyses today.

In fact, semen testing methods today are much more sophisticated and accurate than they were even 20 years ago and so it may be unreasonable to compare results based on what may be very different criteria. There is no evidence that subfertility has increased over the past 40 years, and although sperm *counts* may be reduced, sperm *function* may not have been affected. The drop in the birth-rate is more likely to be attributable to modern contraceptive methods and the availability of abortion. It has been suggested that pollution, which affects foetal development, may be responsible for a decrease in sperm counts, but this remains to be clinically proven.

Other factors may also have contributed to a rise in the number of couples seeking medical help for subfertility. The increased use of contraceptive methods, such as the IUD, or coil, in the last 20 years, may have added to the problem, as this may affect subsequent fertility by increasing the risk of pelvic inflammatory disease. There is no evidence that taking the Pill increases the risk of subsequent infertility, although it may take a few more months for fertility to return to normal after stopping the Pill than it might after using a barrier method of contraception.

There has been an increase in the incidence of sexually transmitted disease over the past 30 or so years, and more men and women are likely to have had more sexual partners than might have been the case 30 years ago, increasing the opportunity of transmitting or contracting infections such as pelvic inflammatory disease, which may lead to blockage of the Fallopian tubes and subsequent infertility.

Publicity given to modern fertility treatments may also encourage more couples to seek assistance, where previously they may have been prepared to accept their situation. The considerable reduction in babies available for adoption over the last 20 years has also forced more couples to try every possible clinical method to enable them to have their own child.

In general, couples who have not conceived within two years will require medical investigation. With the treatments available today, more than two-thirds of these couples can be helped to have a family of their own. Specialists in the field of human reproduction believe that, if all the current medical technology were available to *every* subfertile couple, regardless of cost and other constraints, only about 4 per cent of couples would remain involuntarily childless.

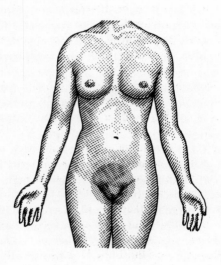

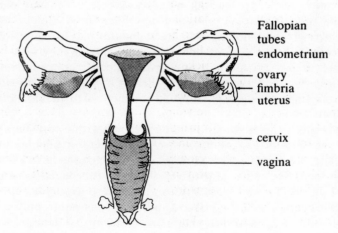

Fallopian tubes
endometrium
ovary
fimbria
uterus
cervix
vagina

Figure 1. *The female reproductive system.*

♀ ♂ *How does pregnancy occur?*

In order to understand the causes of subfertility, it is necessary to understand how pregnancy occurs.

For conception to take place, healthy sperm must find their way to the egg and fertilize it. The fertilized egg must then make its way to the womb, which must be prepared to accept it (see Figure 1). Egg and sperm production are controlled by a complicated system of hormone release.

The average woman produces an egg (ovulates) towards the middle of her menstrual cycle, approximately 14 days before her period is due. It is normal to produce one egg only, each month from one of the two ovaries.

At birth, the average woman already has her full complement of eggs, around 400 000. This number will have fallen considerably by the time she reaches puberty, and will continue to fall throughout her life. After puberty, hormones (chemical messengers released into the blood stream) cause around 20 eggs in the ovaries to start to develop each month, of which only 1 will ripen fully. The remaining eggs that started to develop will degenerate.

Each egg develops inside a fluid-filled sac called a follicle. The fluid bathes and nourishes the egg and the follicle grows as the egg matures. Just prior to ovulation the dominant follicle measures around 20–25 mm. In response to hormonal stimulus a small opening appears in the follicle and the fluid containing the egg is released from the ovary (ovulation) and picked up by the fingerlike projections (fimbriae) at the end of the corresponding Fallopian tube and propelled through the tube towards the womb. During this time further hormones prepare the womb lining to receive the fertilized egg. Intercourse should occur just prior to ovulation if pregnancy is to follow, as the woman's body is most receptive at this time.

The average man produces many millions of sperm, which can be ejaculated at any time. Sperm are produced in the testicles (see Figure 2). The process of sperm production is ongoing, taking around 70–74 days, starting at puberty.

Sperm develop in tiny tubes known as seminiferous tubules, which collect into another larger tube called the epididymis. When they are fully developed, they pass from the testicles into the penis via a tube known as the vas deferens. Semen is a fluid produced by the prostate gland and other glands to carry and nourish the sperm. When the penis becomes erect and orgasm occurs, muscles at the base of the

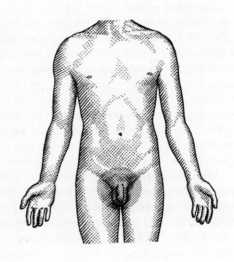

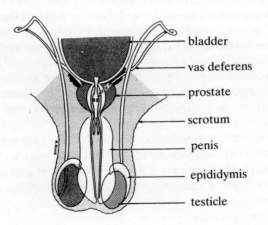

bladder
vas deferens
prostate
scrotum
penis
epididymis
testicle

Figure 2. *The male reproductive system.*

penis pump spurts of seminal fluid carrying millions of sperm through a channel opening at the end of the penis known as the urethra.

During intercourse, the erect penis is inserted into the vagina where sperm are deposited when the man ejaculates. Each sperm has to swim through the neck of the womb (cervix) into the womb itself, then into the Fallopian tubes. Of the many millions of sperm deposited in the vagina, many will die. The strongest sperm will meet the egg in one of the Fallopian tubes and just one of them will fertilize it. It is not necessary for a woman to experience an orgasm for her to conceive.

The ripe egg that has been released into the Fallopian tube is capable of being fertilized for 12–24 hours following ovulation, after which it will degenerate. Sperm may reach the Fallopian tubes only minutes after ejaculation, but they may survive for three or four days or even longer. This means that successful fertilization can occur if intercourse takes place 1 or even 2 days before ovulation, but fertilization is unlikely if intercourse occurs more than 24 hours after ovulation. Thus, in any normal cycle, the opportunity for conception is likely to be around three to four days around the time of ovulation.

The lining of the Fallopian tubes is covered with special cells, called cilia, and these carry the fertilized egg towards the womb about five days after ovulation, Around seven days after fertilization, the fertilized egg, or pre-embryo, will become firmly implanted within the thickened lining (endometrium) of the womb and start to develop.

If, for any reason this process fails, at any stage, and conception does not occur, the thickened lining of the womb will be shed and the woman will have her period, usually between 12 and 16 days after ovulation.

The process of fertilization and conception relies on a network of chemical messengers or hormones, which stimulate the various male and female organs to produce sperm and eggs. Hormones are also responsible for preparing the womb for pregnancy and sustaining the embryo after conception.

In summary, there are four key factors that affect fertility:

- egg production
- sperm production
- the absence of any barriers that would prevent sperm meeting egg
- the right conditions for the fertilized egg to implant in the womb.

Any failure in any one of these processes will lead to subfertility.

Human fertility is – in spite of the overpopulation of the planet – an inefficient process. It is known that partners who are both fertile have only a 20–25 per cent chance of achieving a pregnancy each month, so, even when there are no known difficulties, pregnancy is not guaranteed.

♀ ♂ *Is there a problem?*

If you haven't conceived and you are beginning to be concerned, the first thing to do is consult your GP. He or she can check your medical histories for any possible problems, conduct a simple physical examination of you both, and confirm that ovulation is occurring regularly. Your doctor will be looking to confirm that the periods occur regularly, every 25–35 days, your general health is good, you have intercourse at the right time in the cycle, and that neither partner has any medical history that might affect fertility.

Your GP may not instigate any investigations if he or she feels you have not been trying long enough. A rule of thumb you could use is based on the age of the female partner. If she's under 30 years old you should see your GP soon if you haven't conceived after 18 months of regular, unprotected intercourse. If she's aged between 30 and 35, see your doctor after 12 to 18 months of trying, and after 12 months if she's over 35.

Secondary Subfertility

It is particularly distressing and perplexing if, after conceiving normally in the past, you find you are unable to complete your family. This is known as secondary subfertility and can be just as distressing as primary subfertility, as the feelings of lack of control, loss and grief are just as intense. These are exacerbated by additional pressures from your child to have a sibling when all his or her friends have little brothers or sisters, and the reluctance to press your case when you know you are so lucky to have even one child.

Many couples who find they are unable to have a further child, whether it is a second or even a third, feel guilty about seeking help when they are so aware that access to treatment even for couples with no children is so restricted. None the less, if pregnancy has not followed unprotected intercourse after one to two years it is still important to seek help from your GP.

Age and fertility

Doctors have estimated that normally fertile women aged up to 25 years require on average 2–3 months to conceive compared with women over 35 who require 6 months or longer. In research conducted in Bristol, couples with unexplained infertility were assessed and the time taken for them to conceive, following treatment, was measured in relation to the age of the woman. It can be seen that there was little difference between those women aged between under 25 years and 35, but after 35 there is a marked drop in the number of women conceiving. Similar results have also been found when considering couples undergoing donor insemination treatment.

There are a number of reasons for age being an important factor in female fertility. Whereas men produce new sperm all the time, women are born with their full complement of eggs, and the number

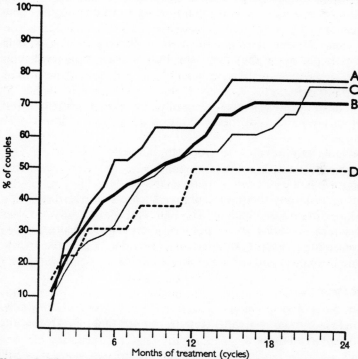

Figure 3. *The cumulative rates of conception following treatment of couples with unexplained subfertility related to the age of the woman: line A denotes under 25, line B 25–29, line C 30–34, line D 35 and over.*

gradually reduces throughout their lives. Her eggs have been subjected to the full effects of her environment and, when *she* is older, the *eggs* are older, too. This may mean that more of her eggs are abnormal, which may lead to abnormal embryos, which fail to implant or are more likely to miscarry.

As a woman becomes older, there is a chance that more of her cycles will produce no viable egg, and there is also a greater likelihood of endometriosis and fibroids (see page 66). There is some evidence that the endometrium of an older woman may be less receptive than when she is younger, which may also reduce the chances of an embryo successfully implanting. Age only begins to be a factor in male fertility when a man is around 60 years old, and very little research has been done in this area.

As the age of the female partner can make a considerable difference to the outcome of treatment, coupled with the fact that there may be some delay before appropriate treatment within the NHS can commence, it is important to register your concerns about your fertility with your GP promptly.

See your GP straight away if any of the following criteria apply to you or your partner as they may contribute to a delay in conceiving.

♀ *For the woman*

- You have erratic, irregular, scanty, or absent periods, your periods are painful for their full duration or you find intercourse painful.
- You have had previous treatment for cancer.
- You have already lost a pregnancy.
- You have had pelvic inflammatory disease.
- You have had any abdominal surgery, such as removal of appendix or have previously had an IUD or coil fitted. Any invasive procedure involving the abdomen or reproductive organs may increase the possibility of infection, which might give rise to scar tissue formation and subsequent tubal damage.

♂ *For the man*

- You have had previous treatment for cancer, undescended testicles, or mumps orchitis (that is, mumps that has affected the testicles) in adulthood.

♀ ♂ *For both partners*

- You or your partner have had sexually transmitted disease, are considerably overweight or underweight, smoke or drink alcohol to excess.

♀ ♂ *What can you do for yourself?*

Before doing anything else, check about one important thing. German measles, known as rubella, can cause serious congenital abnormalities in a child whose mother contracts the disease in early pregnancy. It is important that your doctor checks for immunity to rubella before you try for a baby or treatment commences.

There are several practical things you can do for yourself that will do you good and help improve your chances of becoming pregnant. If you are unfit or under stress, your fertility might be affected. There is some dispute about the effects of stress on fertility, although it is known that emotional and physical stress can result, very rarely, in a condition known as hyperprolactinaemia. This condition in women affects the release of hormones essential to ovulation and can lead to amenorrhoea, that is where ovulation stops and so pregnancy is impossible.

Many couples find that the spotlight of investigations, the pressure to make love to order, and the strength of emotions they both feel about their subfertility can lead to a reluctance on the part of one or the other, or indeed both, to make love at all.

Subfertility itself is a considerably stressful condition, so it is helpful, where possible, to reduce or manage other sources of stress effectively at this stage.

Although it seems that many couples have children so easily, without even trying, regardless of their health and fitness, you can take a look at your life-style and see if there are any ways you can both improve your general fitness, either as a preparation for pregnancy and parenthood or to help you through the rigours of treatment and investigations, or just to help you feel better about yourselves.

There is no evidence that your life-style is likely to have any bearing on your fertility problems, but if you feel that it might be helpful, or you just want to do something positive, you might like to ask yourselves some questions. Do you eat a balanced diet? This should include unrefined food, such as wholemeal bread, fresh fruit and vegetables. Do you take regular exercise? This may only mean a brisk walk two or three times a week, but even better are swimming, cycling, or any active sport performed regularly as this will help you become and stay fit. Too much exercise, however, may reduce fertility in women. Some female athletes have been known to stop ovulating altogether.

Women who are seriously underweight may stop ovulating or find that their menstrual cycle is likely to be erratic. Conversely, doctors may find it difficult to conduct some of the important diagnostic tests on women who are very overweight and serious obesity may exacerbate a condition such as poly cystic ovarian syndrome.

A report published in the United States has suggested that women trying to become pregnant who drink more than four cups of coffee a day are half as likely to succeed as those who drink only small amounts of coffee, although this has not been substantiated in any other reports to date. Further recent reports have also linked even moderate caffeine intake with an increased risk of miscarriage.

Do either of you smoke? Smoking has been shown to reduce the chance of conceiving, increase the risk of miscarriage and reduce growth of the foetus during pregnancy, so that the baby is likely to be small at birth. Most women would naturally wish to give up smoking when they become pregnant, so why not start now?

Sperm volume and quality may be adversely affected by smoking, so it is equally important that both partners cut down or stop smoking. Furthermore, research conducted in Bristol has demonstrated that even passive smoking can reduce fertilization rates in IVF patients. Another advantage of giving up smoking is that you can save the money you would have spent on cigarettes and put it into your 'baby fund'!

How much alcohol do you drink? If you drink more than the equivalent of two glasses of wine or spirits, three times a week, you may be drinking too much. Some recent research suggested a link between drinking even moderate amounts of alcohol and a diminished fertilization rate in women. Most women cut down their alcohol intake during pregnancy so why not cut down now? There is evidence that alcoholism, marijuana, and hard drugs, such as morphine and heroin, can give rise to both impotence and infertility in men, and marijuana is known to affect hormone secretion in women, which may lead to ovulation disorders.

If either of you are taking any medication, do discuss this with your doctor. Some drugs given to women may prevent pregnancy, and some should be avoided during pregnancy as they may harm the baby. Other drugs prescribed for a variety of conditions may impair male fertility, but your doctor should be aware of this, and, in most cases, there will be alternative drugs that can be prescribed. Avoid any drugs not prescribed by your doctor.

Finally, sperm production may be affected by contact with certain chemicals a man may encounter through his occupation, Most employers should be aware of any health hazards posed by working conditions, and they have an obligation to make this known to employees. Occupational health or health and safety at work officials can advise you, as can your doctor. There are reported incidences of prolonged exposure to certain pesticides, such as DBCP (dibromo-chloropropane) in manufacture, causing infertility in men, and it is thought that the lead Romans used to sweeten their food and wine was responsible for a decline in male fertility, playing a not insignificant part in the fall of the Roman Empire!

Everyone is aware of the effects of stress on physical well-being. If either of you is under stress, anxiety over subfertility is an added burden. If you are able to analyse the cause of your stress, such as work or family problems, you may be able to address and overcome it.

Sometimes a vicious circle develops in which a woman finds herself in a job she dislikes but she knows that she will be able to leave once she is pregnant. Every period sees her facing another month in a job she doesn't enjoy. In this situation it might be worth looking for a job that would be more satisfying, perhaps voluntary work with less financial reward or, perhaps, giving up work altogether, if she can afford it.

If you do embark on what may be a long road of investigations and treatment, often conducted at clinics some distance from home, you may feel that you cannot give your all to your career while you have to keep dashing off for appointments. If employers are unsympathetic or unaware of the reasons for your frequent absences, this may add to the pressure for you to give up work, particularly if you had intended to give up work when you started your family.

Women who become pregnant after giving up work are unlikely to be eligible for maternity pay. Similarly, just because a woman longs to be a mother, that need not necessarily mean she should give up work after her baby arrives. For her to receive full maternity leave and benefits she would have to keep on working well into her pregnancy and plan to return after the baby is born.

Alongside the anger and guilt many individuals experience with subfertility is a feeling of depression. This is often associated with a thoughtless remark from a friend, relative, or even a total stranger, who is probably completely unaware of the situation. Many couples find it helpful to share their experience with others in the same position.

There are two main national support groups – CHILD and ISSUE (The National Fertility Association Ltd) – see page 144 for their addresses. While you may not wish to join either group, you may find it helpful to talk with someone who understands how you feel. It is also comforting to read the experiences of others who have felt the same frustration and pain as you in the regular newsletters sent to members, and, purely from a practical point of view, it is good to learn about new developments in your area from local support groups. CHILD and ISSUE campaign actively for improved services for the subfertile and your support is invaluable to them.

It is important to seek professional help if you feel that your sex life is not all it might be. It is important that the penis penetrates the vagina and deposits semen deep within the vagina through ejaculation during male orgasm. It is not necessary for the female partner to experience orgasm in order to conceive. As many as 6 per cent of subfertile couples included in a recent study were not achieving penetration or making love at the right time for conception to occur. Your local Relate office or your family doctor will be able to advise you.

Your sexual relationship may come under considerable stress at times, particularly if you are monitoring ovulation – that is, you have assessed the time when the ovary is most likely to release its egg and you make love at the right time to coincide with it. Many couples find it difficult or impossible to 'make love to order' at this time. This takes the spontaneity and joy out of lovemaking.

Quite a few couples experiment with different positions during lovemaking or just after because they believe this will enhance their chances of conception. These may include the woman lifting her bottom on to a pillow after intercourse to prevent the sperm draining out. However, providing the penis deposits the sperm inside the vagina, there is no evidence that any particular position will improve the chances of success. Similarly, although some of the seminal fluid is likely to run out of the vagina following intercourse, the sperm are able to penetrate cervical mucus very quickly, regardless of position.

♀ Ovulation prediction

One key way in which you can maximize the chances of conceiving is to time intercourse to coincide with ovulation. There are only a few days during each cycle when an egg is ripe for fertilization.

A 'cycle' is the time between the start of one period and the start of the next. To count the days of a cycle, start with the first day of menstrual bleeding; this is day 1. Continue counting the days until the first day of the next period, when you will return to day 1 again. The length of the cycle is the number of days that have elapsed before the period begins again. An average cycle lasts approximately 28 days, although there can be considerable variations in the length of a normal cycle.

There are varying views about the timing and frequency of intercourse, but the general consensus of opinion is that couples should make love at least every other day during the time when ovulation is expected to occur. Sperm are capable of fertilizing an egg up to 48 hours after ejaculation, some even longer, and an egg can be fertilized for up to 24 hours after ovulation, which gives a window of around 3 days in the cycle during which time intercourse must take place.

You may feel happier if you have relaxed and enjoyable sex several times around the predicted time of ovulation rather than pinpoint ovulation and 'perform' there and then as most couples find this, at best, inconvenient and, at worst, simply impossible. But whether your normal pattern is to make love once a week, once a fortnight, or once a month, if you are trying to conceive, you must make love at least once during the three days that ovulation is expected.

Regular sex during the remainder of the cycle is more likely to improve male fertility than to impair it, so it is not advisable to abstain for the rest of the month until ovulation time comes around again. Sperm only have a given life cycle, so if you abstain for the rest of the month, the semen is likely to contain a higher proportion of dead sperm. So, while the quantity may be greater, the quality is unlikely to improve.

In a regular 28-day cycle, ovulation will normally take place 12–14 days before the period. A normal cycle can vary from three to six weeks, but if the period is irregular, scanty, or even absent, ovulation may not be occurring at all. Even when the period occurs regularly, every 28 days, this is not necessarily a definite indication of ovulation.

If you keep a record of your menstrual cycle over a period of months, you can assess those days when ovulation is most likely to occur. By counting the number of days in each cycle and subtracting 14, you will arrive at the earliest and latest possible times of ovulation over the previous months. For example, if over the previous 6 months the shortest cycle was 26 days and the longest was 30 days, by subtracting 14 from each total, you can estimate that, over a 6-month period, ovulation occurred between day 12 and day 16 (that is 26 − 14 = 12 and 30 − 14 = 16). The chance of conception is best, then, if you make love every day or every other day, starting on day 11, the day before ovulation, until day 16.

There are a number of ways in which you can determine both whether and when ovulation is occurring.

Temperature charts Many of the leading fertility consultants feel that temperature charts as a reliable indication of ovulation can be misleading as there are many other reasons for temperature rising, and, as the temperature has to be taken every single day, they also serve as a constant reminder, every morning, every day that you are subfertile. None the less, they continue to be offered to many couples as a first line of investigation.

One consultant recently wrote that he felt that temperature charts were just a way in which doctors can 'fob patients off giving them [the doctors] a six-month breathing space when the woman might get pregnant normally'. The principle behind the temperature chart is that a very slight temperature rise occurs after ovulation. Your doctor may give you a chart on which the woman records her temperature first thing every morning. This is sometimes called 'basal body temperature' (BBT).

This might be a worthwhile test for one month or so, as an indicator of ovulation, rather than a prompt for intercourse, but, for the reasons already outlined, many couples find that it places undue pressure on them to make love to order, particularly first thing in the morning when they both may have to rush out to work. The charts only indicate that ovulation has occurred *after* the event, leaving only a very brief 'window of opportunity' of less than 24 hours during which the egg can be fertilized.

Ovulation predictor kits There are a number of these kits on the market today. They offer a simple method of predicting ovulation just before it happens by detecting a subtle change in hormone levels. These tests, which are available from most high street chemist shops, can be conducted at home. They take about 5–20 minutes and are relatively simple to use, although they can be quite expensive.

Most of the kits contain enough material to test over a number of days. Using sophisticated technology a sample of urine is tested with a chemical reagent that will indicate the stage of ovulation by means of a colour change.

The reagent measures an increase in the luteinizing hormone (LH). This hormone has an important part to play in ovulation. The ovary is stimulated by a hormone known as follicle stimulating hormone (FSH). As the name suggests, this hormone causes follicles, containing eggs, to develop. As the follicles begin to grow, they secrete oestrogen. The effect of this oestrogen is to cause a falling off in the level of FSH, and, subsequently, all but the most dominant follicle fail to develop any further.

The dominant follicle continues to secrete oestrogen which eventually triggers a sudden release of LH from the pituitary gland. LH causes the egg in the dominant follicle to mature and, around 36 hours after the beginning of what is known as the LH surge, ovulation occurs.

Detecting the LH surge is, then, a very precise method of timing ovulation, giving you up to 36 hours' warning that ovulation is imminent. When the level of LH in urine rises, the test indicator will change colour.

Many specialists are so satisfied with the accuracy of these tests that they are being used to predict ovulation for many of the special subfertility treatments that rely on accurate timing for their success.

If periods are regular, it might be a simple matter to judge which is the best day to test. With irregular periods, however, you may need to test on a number of successive days to achieve an indication of ovulation. This may mean buying another test kit.

Such kits are very useful in that they can help show not only when ovulation is occurring, but that it is occurring at all. There may be small margins of error, however, with such tests and so, if after repeated testing you are unable to identify ovulation, you should consult your GP, who will be able to confirm the occurrence of ovulation through special blood tests.

Before buying an ovulation predictor test, talk to your local pharmacist who will be happy to advise you in its use. A pharmacist, like your own doctor will be able to offer you confidential, professional advice about how and when to use these test kits, as well as explaining the differences between various available brands.

Testing cervical mucus There is a natural method of predicting ovulation. This involves checking for a sticky mucus secreted by the cervix. The mucus can be thick, white or pale yellow, and sticky. As ovulation approaches, this mucus becomes more copious, clear and elastic. Some women may notice a slight discharge on their pants at this time.

If some of this mucus is collected when it becomes noticeable and stretched between two fingers, it will stretch to a length of 10–12.5 cm (4–5 in) when ovulation is near.

Many women find this a simple and useful method of predicting ovulation while others find it messy and unpleasant.

There are some women who are able to ascertain that they are ovulating without the need for any form of testing. This is because they experience discomfort towards the middle of their cycle for a day or so (this is known as mittelschmerz, meaning middle of the month), just before the egg is released from the ovary, along with some symptoms, such as breast tenderness and sometimes increased libido.

♂ *Home sperm testing*

There are now kits available with which men can test their own sperm. They work on the principle of a colour change – red indicating a positive result and purple a negative one, with various degrees of shading in between, to indicate that there are motile (healthy) sperm present. These tests may prove reassuring if the response is good, but there may be some inherent problems with such assessments.

In the event that the result is not good, you may feel very stressed and concerned, and, in the absence of qualified medical staff to interpret the results and indicate the next course of action as well as to provide counselling support, you may both feel quite isolated.

If the result appears promising there may still be a difficulty, as the test is designed to indicate the *presence* of motile sperm in quantities higher than 20 millions per millilitre of semen, not the *quality* of those present. The quality and the way sperm move is as important as the number present and so an indication that all is well may give a false picture. It is also possible that signs of infection in the semen may give a false positive result.

This test may be particularly useful when assessing the outcome of vasectomy reversal, but, as it is quite expensive and as it is unlikely that any doctor will rely on the results from such a test without conducting further semen analyses at a reliable laboratory, its usefulness may be limited.

♀ ♂ *Complementary medicine*

In addition to the practical methods of helping to maximize your fertility and prepare for pregnancy that have been suggested, you may find it helpful to consider some forms of complementary medicine.

There is increasing interest in the role of alternative or holistic medicine. This takes many forms, all of which work on the principle of treating the human body as a whole rather than an organ or disease in isolation.

Few practitioners of alternative medicine are recognized by the NHS, unless they are also qualified in orthodox medicine. In general, alternative medicine is viewed with some scepticism by NHS doctors.

There are, though, many different forms of complementary medicine that, if practised by a reputable practitioner, may be helpful. Some may make claims that they can cure some conditions related to subfertility, such as endometriosis, but it has not been possible to substantiate these.

Whatever form such treatment may take, all may prove to be soothing and helpful, although there is no published evidence to support the argument that any of these therapies will be successful in overcoming fertility problems.

Such treatment may make you feel relaxed and fit, and you will be encouraged to enjoy a good diet and a calmer life-style. It is unlikely that any irreversible action will be taken and you may, for whatever reason, become pregnant.

3
What happens next?

Introduction

This chapter deals with the processes by means of which a diagnosis can be achieved. The diagnosis itself is covered in the next chapter.

Once you have begun to worry about your fertility you should consult your family doctor. Research has shown that 90 per cent of all fertile couples will conceive within one year. If, however, you have left starting a family until later in life you may feel anxious after only six months without success.

Your doctor will have your medical records and can obtain your partner's records, with appropriate consent, if you do not attend the same doctor. These may highlight any immediate cause for concern.

♀ ♂ *Your family doctor*

Too many couples report a lack of urgency in the medical management of their subfertility, and that they need to maintain constant pressure on their doctors to get appropriate attention. Your doctor may tell you to wait a few months before deciding whether or not to begin investigations or treatment. You may be content to wait or you may find that those few months bring further stress and unhappiness as each period arrives. While your doctor can initiate some preliminary investigations, you may need to be referred to a specialist clinic. The provision of specialist services within the NHS is poor and waiting lists can be lengthy, so the sooner you consult your doctor and they start investigations the better.

In 1992, The Royal College of Obstetricians and Gynaecologists Fertility Committee produced a report entitled 'Infertility: Guidelines for practice'. It was prepared for doctors as a 'statement of good practice' in this area.

One of the recommendations made in the report is that couples who are concerned about their fertility should be seen by their GP, 'regardless of the duration of the infertility'. The report also notes that 'the general practitioner/secondary referral interface, was thought to be amenable to improvement'!

Before going to see your doctor, ask if it is possible to have a longer appointment than normal. Inform the doctor why you are coming. If your doctor doesn't have a receptionist, write a note directly to him or her. You will not feel comfortable discussing such a deeply personal and important issue in a hurry and you would almost certainly be asked to return again for a longer consultation.

In many areas, there are group practices where, although you have signed on with one doctor, you can actually have a consultation with any of the partners. The practice nurse or the receptionist will probably know if any of the doctors has a particular interest in subfertility.

In the first instance, your family doctor will check to verify immunity against German measles (rubella). This is because German measles can cause severe foetal abnormality if contracted in the early stages of pregnancy.

Your doctor will need to know what has been happening and need to ask questions about both your medical histories, your sex life, and how long you have been trying to become pregnant. You may find this embarrassing, but your doctor is specially trained to help you, and the interview is likely to be far less traumatic than you may expect. Any information you give to your doctor will be treated in the strictest confidence.

Your doctor will need the following information about you and your partner:

- age, occupation, nature and stability of your relationship
- past medical history and relevant family medical history
- use of alcohol, drugs, and tobacco
- details of previous contraception and previous pregnancies
- frequency of periods
- frequency of intercourse.

Your doctor is likely to carry out a brief physical examination of both partners (if you attend the first appointment together) to eliminate the presence of any obvious abnormality.

The drive to have a family may sometimes be greater in one partner than the other, and it is perfectly natural to feel some embarrassment about discussing such a personal matter with your doctor. Either partner may feel that the failure to achieve pregnancy is a reflection of their own sexuality. This is not the case, but, if one partner refuses, it is impossible to force them to seek investigation against their will.

If the solution to your problem is simple – such as the timing of intercourse or a simple change in life-style – it might never be necessary for both of you to see the doctor. In the event of further investigations and treatment being required, however, it is most important for both partners to be involved. After all, you will both share the responsibility of parenthood.

The importance of your relationship with your doctor cannot be overestimated. If you become pregnant, your doctor will help you through your pregnancy, and care for your child's health. You will need even more support from your doctor if you are to embark on the long road of subfertility investigations.

Changing your doctor

Some family doctors will respond to your concern about having a family by reassuring you, telling you simply to go away and keep trying. A growing number will, however, share your concern and start to help you straight away. If you feel your doctor does not appreciate the depth of your concern, make another appointment after a month or so, particularly if you have been trying for a baby for more than two years. If you appear before him/her every month to share your grief at the arrival of yet another period, he/she will soon get the message and start investigations!

In the rare event that you feel you do not have the support of your doctor, and repeated visits have been unhelpful, you may decide to change your doctor.

This is not particularly easy as you would need to find another doctor prepared to take you. It is possible to find out if another doctor in your area is particularly sympathetic by contacting your local CHILD or ISSUE contact. If another doctor is recommended who practises in your area, write and ask to be put on the list, explaining your situation.

You can also ask for help from a family planning clinic, some of which run special subfertility clinics, but you will still need a letter of referral from your GP before you can be referred on to a specialist.

♀ ♂ The clinic appointment

If your doctor has decided to refer you to a specialist for further investigation, that specialist is most likely to be a gynaecologist. There are approximately 1000 gynaecology consultants in the United Kingdom. Their work includes management of a wide variety of women's conditions from puberty to menopause and after, including pregnancy, contraception, urinary problems, childbirth, and cancer.

The management of subfertility is only a small part of the work of the gynaecologist and some would rather not deal with it at all. This may be because they do not have the staff and equipment to diagnose and treat subfertility well, or perhaps they do not have the facilities to assess both partners together.

Occasionally, if your medical history suggests it, your doctor may refer one or both of you to an endocrinologist, who specializes in the study of male fertility, or a urologist, who deals with the genito-urinary tract, including the male reproductive system.

The working party of The Royal College of Obstetricians and Gynaecologists has recommended the creation of a new sub-speciality of reproductive medicine, which would include infertility, covering the needs of both men and women equally, but there are very few such centres in the country and some areas are particularly poorly served. It is likely then, that your first clinic appointment will take place at the nearest hospital where there is a gynaecology department. This is called secondary referral – that is, your doctor has referred you to a second doctor or clinic.

A good clinic will send you an information sheet along with details of your first appointment, telling you a little about the clinic and what you can expect to happen at your first and subsequent visits. You may also receive a questionnaire to complete about your medical history. If, following referral, you do not hear from the clinic for some weeks or months, telephone to check that they have received your doctor's referral letter. It is not uncommon for these letters to go astray and this may delay your appointment time.

The subfertility clinic, if there is one, may be combined with a general gynaecology out-patients clinic, although sometimes, regrettably, you may also be expected to wait alongside antenatal patients and those seeking a termination of their pregnancies.

Although the appointment may be in the woman's name, it is reasonable to expect that both partners will attend. There is no point in investigating one partner alone as problems may be found in either or both partners. A good clinic will treat both partners as a couple, but there have been many reports from male partners who feel that they are treated as though they are incidental to the proceedings or even invisible. This is difficult to overcome, but such feelings should be conveyed to the staff of the clinic at the time or following the appointment, in writing.

WHAT HAPPENS NEXT?

You should expect to be seen, on the first occasion, by the Consultant or Registrar, who will have a record of your previous medical history from your doctor. You can help the clinic if you go armed with the following information:

- dates and details of any previous operations, pregnancies or illnesses
- results and dates of any cervical smear tests performed
- results of any tests your GP may have conducted.

It is often helpful to keep a diary, marking the first day of menstrual periods over the past 6–12 months, and the days on which you had intercourse during that time.

It can be difficult to share such intimate information with a doctor who is new to you. Many patients find that, at subsequent clinic attendances they never see the same doctor twice, so they have to go over the same ground again, each time. It might be an idea to keep a brief note of your investigations and treatment starting at this point and keep this with you for future appointments.

When you see the specialist, make sure you have a note of any questions you want to ask them. Too often, patients feel overawed by the specialist and forget all the things they wanted to ask. You will have waited a long time for this appointment and may have to wait a long time for the next, so make the most of your time with the doctor.

If you find that you don't understand anything the doctor tells you, ask for an explanation. Some doctors tend to use long, unfamiliar words to describe something simple, so make sure you know what they're talking about! Subfertility treatment has given rise to a considerable number of acronyms, such as GIFT, DIPSI and SUZI, that spelt out, become even more incomprehensible. If you don't understand, ask! If you still don't understand ask for it in writing! Most good clinics will have clear, written instructions on most procedures; those that don't should be encouraged to do so.

The objective of the clinic appointment is to establish why you have not yet conceived. Ideally, once you have been referred you should be seen within three to six months, and investigations to reach a diagnosis should be complete within three to six months of the first clinic appointment. This is more likely to happen if your GP refers you to a clinic where the consultant gynaecologist is particularly interested in subfertility, although some specialist clinics have considerable waiting lists for a first appointment.

After initial investigations are complete, the clinic will make another appointment – hopefully within six to eight weeks – to review their findings and discuss the next step.

Reaching a diagnosis

In order to arrive at a diagnosis, the clinic will begin a series of investigations. The order in which these are done may vary and, in the event that an early diagnosis is made, not all tests will be performed.

These tests include:

- the collection of a full medical history from both partners
- tests for female partner to confirm ovulation
- semen analysis
- laparoscopy and dye
- hysterosalpingogram.

Results from these preliminary investigations will provide a diagnosis for 75 per cent of couples, and, depending on the results of these tests, further investigations may be required before appropriate treatment can be recommended.

Ideally, it should be possible for all preliminary tests to be completed within three to six months, although many patients at clinics not specifically dedicated to the management of subfertility find that they undergo a few tests followed by a lengthy wait before the next appointment. If you leave the clinic without a date for your follow-up appointment, or without any clear idea of what the next step will be, don't leave it too long before telephoning to make sure that your notes or test results have not been mislaid.

Medical history

The clinic doctor will ask you both about your previous medical histories – the time you have spent trying for a family and a general picture of your present health and life-style. He will also need to ask whether either of you have ever had any sexually transmitted disease or whether either partner has proven fertility through a previous relationship.

One woman told of her embarrassment when a doctor asked her, in the presence of her partner, how many sexual partners she had previously had! While this may have been relevant information that could have helped the doctor to build up an accurate picture of her reproductive medical history, it was not the kind of information she wanted to share with her partner!

Doctors may have questions they need to ask both partners that might cause embarrassment to the other. The opportunity for them to do this discreetly should present itself when either partner is being examined or perhaps when the man goes to arrange his semen analysis. Sometimes, however, the opportunity doesn't arise or the doctor fails to realize that the subject may be sensitive.

If this should happen, there are two ways to handle it: either to answer honestly to the embarrassment of both yourself and your partner, or to give a vague answer and contact the doctor later with the appropriate information. This is not an unusual occurrence, so, if it happens, you might also like to let the doctor know how insensitive you felt his questioning was.

Don't feel under pressure if you have information which the doctor should have of which your partner may be unaware. You can either write to the doctor with the information, explaining that this is not something you wish to discuss in the presence of your partner, or you can wait until the doctor examines you, when your partner will be outside the room.

A good clinic will have considered your need for an opportunity to talk privately. If it does not happen, you may have to speak discreetly to one of the nursing staff. If either of you feels unhappy about the way you have been treated, do let the clinic staff know as that is the only way care for all patients can improve.

Ideally, the clinic doctor will examine both partners, even if your GP has already done so. The doctor will take several measurements, including height, weight, and blood pressure, and check respiration (breathing) by listening to your chest, and examine your abdomen. These are standard medical procedures to establish that you are both in general good health.

This first appointment is likely to involve an internal examination for the woman, similar to that performed for a cervical smear test. During this examination, the doctor can feel the outline of the uterus and ovaries and detect any obvious physical abnormalities. At the same time, the doctor may collect some of the secretions from around the cervix for analysis. This is usually a painless procedure, which is sometimes referred to as a high vaginal or endocervical swab.

The specimen collected can be tested for the presence of chlamydia or other sign of infection. Chlamydia are pathogens, that is disease-causing organisms similar to bacteria, which may give rise to infection of the Fallopian tubes, causing damage and blockage. It is important to test for this before any treatment commences, particularly as chlamydial infection can exist without causing any symptoms.

Often, at the first consultation, the clinic doctor will examine the genitals of the male partner to eliminate the possibility of there being any obvious abnormality.

Once previous medical histories and physical examinations are complete, the doctor will initiate a series of tests on both partners, some of which will be carried out at the time of the first appointment, some of which will require further attendance, possibly to other hospital departments.

♂ Tests for the man

Semen analysis

The semen analysis, or sperm count as it is sometimes called, is vital before any treatment can be considered for either partner. Even if there is a known reason for your partner not becoming pregnant, it is still important to assess your sperm before any treatment is considered.

Good clinics will require the results of two separate tests before they will venture an opinion on sperm quality. This is because there can be a considerable variation in quality between two samples, owing to simple factors such as a cold or infection during the period when the sperm were produced (the previous 70–74 days).

Producing a semen specimen You may be asked to produce a specimen at home, by masturbation, and take it into the clinic. You will be given a small, sterile pot or, in some cases, be asked to find a suitable clean receptacle at home!

The pots given may be difficult to use if not designed specifically for this purpose. A 30 millilitre pot is commonly used, but is rather small and awkward. An ideal pot will have a capacity of 60 millilitres and a wide top. The object is to obtain a full semen sample (which is generally around 2–5 millilitres), not to fill the pot! Suitable specimen pots are available so if you feel that you may have difficulties using the pot given, ask if the clinic can obtain any that are more suitable.

You should write both your name and your partner's on the pot if the laboratory has not already done so. If they have, check that the name is correct – you don't want it to be confused with anyone else's specimen. The laboratory will ask you to record the date and time of collection of your specimen and the number of days that have elapsed since you last ejaculated. You will be requested to abstain from intercourse or ejaculation for between 48 and 72 hours prior to collection of the specimen in order to provide the best sample.

It is not a good idea to try to collect the sample using coitus interruptus as there is a risk of missing some of the ejaculate, which might give a false test result. Do not use an ordinary condom to collect the semen with a view to emptying it into the pot. Most commercially available condoms contain some form of spermicidal fluid, which will destroy the sperm. The clinic may have a special condom you can use, though, specifically for this purpose.

It is important to protect the specimen from extremes of temperature, until it is handed in to the clinic or laboratory. This is often best achieved by placing the container in a pocket, close to the skin.

When a semen sample is produced, it is a thick, white, viscous fluid. After 20–30 minutes, it becomes less viscous and more liquid, so do not be alarmed if the sample appears to have altered as this is perfectly normal.

If you do not live near enough to the clinic to deliver a specimen produced at home (the specimen needs to be less than two hours old when it is handed in to the laboratory), you may have to produce a specimen at the clinic.

Ideally you will be shown into a private, quiet room to produce your specimen. However, given the constraints of the NHS, you are much more likely to be expected to produce your specimen in the nearest toilet cubicle! This is always difficult and it may be helpful to take a suitable magazine for inspiration, or, if you prefer, you may find it easier if your partner joins you.

It is not unfair to say that some hospital departments are more properly equipped than others to collect and assess semen specimens adequately. If your subsequent treatment programme relies on the result of one or two semen samples, it is vital that they are assessed correctly. It has been suggested by the Royal College of Obstetricians and Gynaecologists' Fertility Committee that the best facilities are likely to be found where there is a tertiary referral centre (that is, a specialist infertility centre), to which you might be referred in the event that your local hospital is unable to help you. This will avoid duplication of investigations and will also ensure that the test results meet the required standards.

No doctor should mind if you ask whether the laboratory to which your sample is being sent is specially equipped to assess semen specimens, but if the clinic you attend is specifically involved with the diagnosis and treatment of subfertility, you are much more likely to get accurate assessments.

The assessment During semen analysis, the volume of seminal fluid and number, movement, and appearance of the sperm is assessed. Specialist clinics might also perform a test to identify any sperm antibodies that might be present. The sperm count is recorded, based on the number of million sperm per millilitre of seminal fluid. This is measured on a microscopic grid system. There are many millions of sperm in each sample – between 20 and 600 million.

The sperm are then studied to see how well they move, as movement is vital in order for them to travel the route to the egg. This is described as sperm motility. Healthy, motile sperm will move forwards in a brisk way. Technicians will also assess the number of white blood cells. An abnormally high level of white blood cells may be an indication of some form of infection. Finally, there is an estimate of the number of abnormal sperm.

A semen analysis will generally give information about the volume, appearance, concentration, motility and morphology of the sample. The normal range for the volume of a sample is generally between 1.5–6 mls, and the concentration or sperm count may range from 20 millions per ml to 120 millions per ml. A typical specimen would demonstrate about 50 per cent motility and around 50 per cent normal forms.

A typical district general hospital without a specialist interest in subfertility is unlikely to have a laboratory producing particularly detailed analyses. When you are given your result do ensure that you have someone at the clinic explain it fully to you.

While the sperm count *is* important, there are other factors that are of equal importance. If there are many millions of sperm, but all of them are deformed and none would be able to swim to the egg, then the count is irrelevant.

The sperm have several functions to perform. They must penetrate cervical mucus and travel through the cervix and uterus to reach the Fallopian tubes. Here one will penetrate the material surrounding the egg, fertilize it, and produce a viable zygote. A zygote is a single fertilized cell formed by the two gametes (the egg and the sperm). The reason that so many sperm are released each time is because very few survive the journey to the egg – perhaps only 100 or 200 – and only one will succeed in fusing with the egg.

There is no such thing as a standard semen sample as volumes may differ considerably and any number of sperm from 20 million to 600 million per millilitre is within normal boundaries.

The sperm consists of a head, body (or midpiece), and tail. The head contains the genetic material, and the midpiece and tail provide the energy for the sperm to reach the egg. The head of the sperm is covered with a layer known as the acrosome, which is involved with the penetration of the egg. The study of the appearance of the sperm is known as morphology, and it is quite within normal boundaries for as many as 40 per cent of a sample to be abnormal.

The movement (motility) and condition (morphology) are important criteria because, no matter how many sperm there are, if they are not moving progresssively, they will not reach the egg, and those that are deformed will not fertilize the egg.

Do not be alarmed at figures like 50 per cent motility or 40 per cent abnormal sperm. These are perfectly normal as, at any given time, some sperm may be immature while some may be dead. It is of much greater concern if *all* the sperm are abnormal or the count is extremely low. Even if the results of repeated samples show a count no greater than 20 million/ml, there is no immediate cause for concern as doctors have proven that as many as 20 per cent of men father children with an average count lower than 20 million/ml.

If you have had an illness such as 'flu in the previous three to four months, do tell the laboratory technician. The sperm released in an ejaculate today were manufactured in the testicles three months ago, so if you were ill at the time there is a possibility that all the sperm will be of very poor quality or there may be none at all. This is why it is so important that the diagnosis is based on the results of more than one test, particularly if the first one is poor.

It is perfectly normal to have three tests conducted at different times with vastly differing results – perhaps as a result of previous illness, a difference in the period of abstinence, or some other factor. In one published trial, the same man produced a specimen once a fortnight over a period of two years. During that time, his sperm volume fluctuated between excellent and almost nil. This proves that no specimen should be looked at in isolation. It has also been proved that many men with poor semen quality (usually considered to be less than 20 million per ml) are capable of fathering children with no difficulty.

In the rare event that there are no sperm whatsoever found in the ejaculate, doctors may run a series of blood tests before requesting further semen samples.

Many clinics will also check a semen sample for signs of infection. If present, antibiotics may be prescribed to clear up the infection and another sample will be tested again later.

Another test, known as the hamster egg penetration test, may possibly be performed. During this, prepared hamster eggs are mixed with prepared sperm to see if penetration occurs. This has some value in assessing the fertilizing capacity of your sperm, but tends to be used primarily for research purposes as some experts believe its clinical usefulness is limited.

♀ Tests for the woman

Confirming ovulation

In the absence of any firm results of previous ovulation monitoring, blood tests may be required to confirm the presence and timing of ovulation.

The menstrual cycle is a complicated process involving several hormones that initiate egg development and growth, while, at the same time, building up the endometrium to prepare for pregnancy. To establish that the menstrual cycle is normal, the doctor will take a blood sample, often on a particular day of your cycle. This may have to be repeated in several cycles.

The blood tests are used to establish that you have a normal hormone profile. The hormones concerned with reproduction are produced by many different organs of the body (known as endocrine glands) such as the pituitary gland situated in the brain, the thyroid gland in the neck, and the ovaries. The hormones assessed include FSH, LH, prolactin, oestrogen, and progesterone.

Doctors may also perform an ultrasound scan of your ovaries and uterus to check ovulation. By means of an ultrasound scan – a painless, safe, and simple procedure – doctors can assess the size and function of the ovary and see whether or not an egg is developing.

You may hear or read about endometrial biopsy, used as an indicator of ovulation. The endometrium is the lining of the womb, and an endometrial biopsy is a procedure during which a small sample of this lining is collected and examined for changes indicative of ovulation. This procedure, usually performed under local anaesthetic, is not in common use today.

Laparoscopy and dye This is a minor operation, performed on the female partner, usually under general anaesthetic. During it, a small operative telescope is inserted into the abdomen through a small incision close to the navel. As with all surgical procedures, there is a small risk of post-operative complication. The laparoscope allows the surgeon to see the ovaries, Fallopian tubes, and the external appearance of the uterus. As it is an invasive operative procedure that might be damaging to a developing foetus, it is important to exclude the possibility of pregnancy, so you may, perversely, be asked to use some form of contraception beforehand, just to make sure.

A coloured dye is introduced into the cervix during the operation. If the pathway through the uterus and Fallopian tubes is clear, the dye can be seen to emerge from the fimbrial ends of each tube. If the dye is slow to emerge from the tubes or fails to emerge, this is an indication that there may be some form of blockage.

Through the laparoscope, the surgeon can identify damage to the tubes, adhesions around the finger-like projections at the end of the tubes (fimbria), which will prevent the eggs being picked up, or adhesions encapsulating the ovaries, preventing the eggs from escaping at all. Adhesions are sheets of tough, fibrous tissue that may occur as a result of infection or previous surgical intervention.

It is also possible to identify endometriosis during laparoscopy. This is a condition in which the lining of the womb spreads outside the womb to cover, perhaps, the Fallopian tubes, ovaries, or other organs within the abdomen.

This operation normally takes about 20–40 minutes, and most patients are allowed home 5 or so hours later. Doctors may prefer some women to be admitted as in-patients for this procedure if there are potential anaesthetic difficulties or if the woman is particularly obese. If you have no one to collect and care for you at home or you live a particularly long way from the clinic, it may be possible for you to stay in hospital for one or two nights after your operation.

Some discomfort – particularly wind – may be experienced in the days following laparoscopy. You should be able to return to work after 48 hours.

This procedure is likely to be the first investigation doctors will conduct if sperm function is found to be within normal ranges and no ovulatory disorders have been identified.

Hysteroscopy and salpingoscopy Hysteroscopy allows a doctor to inspect the inside of the uterus using a fine telescope introduced through the vagina and along the cervical canal. This is particularly useful for identifying abnormalities within the uterus, such as adhesions or fibroids. This might be done as an in-patient procedure under general anaesthetic, or as an out-patient procedure without. It might also be combined with laparoscopy.

Salpingoscopy involves the use of a similar, very fine telescope but this time it is inserted into the ends of the Fallopian tubes during laparoscopy. This allows the doctor to visualize the condition of the lining of the tubes. This information is more commonly ascertained by means of a hysterosalpingogram.

Hysterosalpingogram (HSG) This is an X-ray procedure, during which a radio-opaque dye (that is, one that shows up on X-ray) is introduced into the uterus, via the vagina, while using X-ray visualization. The dye fills the uterus and both Fallopian tubes, spilling out from both ends. The radiologist will take X-ray photographs during the course of the procedure.

This test is valuable as it allows doctors to visualize the inside of the uterus and Fallopian tubes to check for any physical abnormality or blockage. It does not, however, give much indication of the general condition of the Fallopian tubes, which are very thin, delicate tubes lined with fine hairs (cilia) that waft the fertilized egg towards the uterus. This test does not indicate the presence of endometriosis or adhesions around the outside of the tubes and ovaries, and there is a small possibility of false results.

This procedure, which is normally carried out without any anaesthetic or sedation, lasts approximately 20 minutes. It is uncomfortable and, for some women, quite painful. It is advisable to rest for at least 30 minutes afterwards and to make arrangements for someone to accompany you home. Your doctor may prescribe antibiotics for you to take before and afterwards to minimize the risk of infection.

Some patients experience some transient pain or discomfort for two to three days following this procedure, but, in the event of severe pain, always contact your doctor.

You will need to inform the X-ray department of the date of your last period as this procedure can only be carried out when there is no risk of pregnancy. It is considered to be safe during the first 12 days of your cycle.

♀ ♂ *What happens next?*

It should be possible for most of these tests to be completed fairly quickly (within two to three months), after which a decision, based on the findings, can be made about what to do next.

There are a number of possible outcomes:

- a diagnosis of ovulatory disorder is reached
- a diagnosis of sperm disorder is reached
- tubal damage is diagnosed
- no firm diagnosis is reached
- during this time you become pregnant.

Researchers have established the most common causes of infertility in couples to be:

- unexplained infertility   28 per cent
- sperm defects   24 per cent
- ovulatory failure   21 per cent
- tubal damage   14 per cent
- other causes   11 per cent
- endometriosis   6 per cent
- coital failure   6 per cent
- mucus dysfunction   3 per cent
- other male infertility   2 per cent.

The percentages total more than 100 because some couples are found to have more than a single cause for their subfertility. These diagnoses are discussed in detail in the next chapter.

In the event of a diagnosis of ovulatory failure or disorder – that is, the ovaries are not producing an egg regularly – your doctor may initiate treatment to restore ovulation, after which there should be a review of the situation after several months, if pregnancy has not occurred, before further investigation or treatment.

In the event of sperm disorder, you are likely to be referred to an appropriate specialist straight away.

If no clear diagnosis is reached, your doctor is likely to refer you for further investigations.

Over a period of time, further attendance at the clinic will be required to establish and treat the cause of your subfertility. Many couples may be helped by simple treatments, perhaps no more than a course of hormones to regulate erratic periods. Statistically it is known that a number of patients will become pregnant during this time without any treatment. For the remaining couples, however, further appointments, investigations, and treatments will be required.

In most investigations and treatment, it is the woman who will undergo invasive procedures, but whichever partner is subjected to these, it is difficult to watch someone you love suffer pain and disappointment. For this reason, some couples opt out of treatment at an earlier stage than others. This is something only you can decide between you.

The unfortunate fact is that continued hospital appointments may involve waiting considerable lengths of time, during which nothing is being done. Indeed, the waiting list at many dedicated, regional infertility centres for the first appointment may be more than 12 months. A number of reports have criticized the delays involved in clinic appointments and the amount of time couples spend sitting in out-patients departments. This is why it is important that you are referred to an appropriate clinic as soon as possible.

Once the basic investigations to assess ovulation and sperm function have been completed make sure you know both the outcome of the tests and the proposed course of action. If you don't have an appointment with the doctor, phone up and make one, checking with the receptionist or nurse that the doctor will have your results to hand when they see you. It is not unknown for test results and patients' notes to go astray, making your visit a complete waste of time as well as very stressful.

Without being objectionable, it is possible, and sometimes necessary, to be quite assertive about follow-up appointments and investigations. Your GP can be extremely helpful in this instance.

Before treatment can be instigated, a diagnosis must be reached. The tests outlined already will usually be run in tandem, after which it might be possible to eliminate one partner from further investigation. You might want to question any doctor who is prepared to initiate treatment in the absence of any clear diagnosis or in the absence of any semen analyses.

It is to be hoped that a diagnosis will be reached as soon as possible, but few departments have unlimited staff, time, or funding to give a priority to subfertility.

There are a series of additional investigations that may help the clinicians reach a diagnosis. These are itemized next. There is no given order of investigation and not all tests will be necessary.

♀ *Further investigations for the woman*

Ultrasound examination

Ultrasound is now widely used as a diagnostic tool in many areas of medicine. Ultrasound waves are high-frequency sound waves that, when applied to the skin using a probe, will bounce off the internal organs and return to the probe to be interpreted and displayed on a television monitor. This gives the doctor a very accurate picture of the organs and has the advantages of being painless and, as far as we know, safe.

The doctor is able to visualize the uterus and ovaries, and take accurate measurements of developing follicles. If used around the time of ovulation, the doctor can monitor the development and release of the egg, which is a useful method of confirming that ovulation is normal. It can also be used as a crucial means of assessing the effect of superovulation, that is, treatment with special drugs to stimulate the ovaries to produce several eggs at one time.

Through ultrasound, the number of eggs developing in each ovary can be counted and the egg-containing sacs (follicles) can be measured. Ultrasound can also be used to assess the thickening of the endometrium (uterus lining) in response to ovulatory hormones.

Ultrasound examinations can be performed in one of two ways: abdominally or vaginally.

Abdominal ultrasound The ultrasound probe is a small boxlike structure attached to a machine with a display screen like a television monitor. A small amount of lubricant jelly is placed on the abdomen to allow the probe to be moved across the abdomen easily and to maintain close contact with the skin at all times.

In order to obtain the best image, a full bladder is required and this can cause discomfort. If you have been given an appointment for this type of investigation, it is best to plan to arrive about half an hour beforehand. On arrival, drink as much liquid as you can – at least 1–2 pints. Many patients complain if there are delays, as it can be most uncomfortable to sit with a very full bladder for any length of time. It is also very difficult to let just a little out if you become too uncomfortable – unfortunately the floodgates open easily but are rather difficult to close in mid flow! As a result of this, and its cleaner pictures, many doctors favour the use of the vaginal ultrasound probe.

Vaginal ultrasound Another form of ultrasound probe has been developed that does not require a full bladder: the intra-vaginal probe. This fits inside the vagina and has the additional advantage of giving more detailed information about the adjacent organs without pressing down on a straining bladder. To prevent cross-infection, doctors cover the probe with a sterile sheath or condom that is changed after every use.

Most specialist clinics have access to an intra-vaginal probe, but fewer district hospitals will have this facility.

Dilatation and curettage (D & C)

This is a minor operation, usually performed under general anaesthetic. During the operation, a sample of the lining of the uterus (endometrium) is removed for tissue examination to confirm ovulation and to exclude the presence of disease or abnormality.

This may be helpful in detecting fibroids (which are masses of fibrous tissues in the wall of the uterus), and in assessing the state of the endometrium at a given stage in the menstrual cycle. Fibroids are rarely responsible for subfertility and many women with fibroids conceive quite naturally.

Dilatation and curettage is not a common fertility investigation as more information can be obtained by means of laparoscopy, hysteroscopy, ultrasound and hormone measurements.

Tubal insufflation (Rubin's test)

You may have come across references to this procedure, in which air is passed into the Fallopian tubes through the cervix and uterus. It is no longer regarded as an acceptable investigation of tubal status as it is particularly unreliable. It has been superseded by other, more accurate, investigations.

♀ ♂ Combined investigations

The post-coital test

The post coital (post = after, coitus = intercourse) test is performed to demonstrate that sperm are being deposited in the correct place – that is, high in the vagina – during intercourse and that they are able to move forwards in cervical mucus. Some district hospitals will suggest this test quite early on in the management of your subfertility and may not proceed with a semen analysis at all if a good number of healthy sperm are found to be swimming in the mucus.

While this test gives a great deal less information about the sperm volume and quality, it gives important information about the way in which sperm and mucus react when they come into contact.

Mucus is the sticky secretion found around the cervix throughout the menstrual cycle. Mucus plays an important part in conception, as, during the infertile periods of the month, the mucus is naturally hostile to sperm, making it difficult for them to pass through to the womb. As ovulation nears, the appearance of the mucus changes to a clear, elastic fluid, not unlike the white of an egg, as mentioned earlier.

At this stage, mucus is much more welcoming to sperm, allowing easy passage. For this reason, it is important that the post- coital test takes place around the time of ovulation. Under the microscope sperm should normally be seen swimming in the mucus many hours after intercourse. At any other time, the sperm would be seen to be struggling in the mucus, which might give rise to a faulty diagnosis of mucus hostility or poor sperm quality.

For this assessment, you will be requested to have intercourse approximately 6–12 hours prior to the clinic appointment. If you and your partner find it impossible to make love beforehand, inform the clinic as it is pointless to proceed with this test otherwise. The test is a painless procedure whereby the doctor collects a small amount of the mucus from around the cervix. The mucus is smeared onto a glass slide where the doctor can examine it under the microscope.

The doctor is able to see whether or not there are healthy sperm swimming forwards, through the mucus. This fulfils a dual diagnostic role as it gives some indication of both the quality of the sperm and also whether or not the mucus is resistant to the sperm. In mucus resistance, sperm are destroyed by the partner's mucus and so are unable to penetrate the womb, thus never meeting the egg. This is very uncommon except when the timing of the test is incorrect.

If properly timed the absence of motile sperm in the sample more often reflects sperm disorder, therefore some fertility specialists prefer other tests of sperm function that do not need accurately timed mucus collection.

Sperm/mucus crossover interaction test

In this test, sometimes referred to as a sperm/mucus hostility test, sperm and mucus from donors are used in conjunction with sperm and mucus from you and your partner.

If mucus penetration failure has been identified – that is, the sperm were unable to penetrate the mucus – it is valuable to know whether the sperm would be able to penetrate the ovulatory mucus of a donor, as this would indicate whether there is a problem with the sperm or a problem with the mucus. Mucus hostility is relatively rare.

To make these assessments, samples of your sperm and mucus are each mixed with proven samples of donor mucus and donor sperm respectively. The mucus used must be collected during the ovulatory phase of the cycle as during the rest of the cycle mucus is naturally hostile to sperm. The two samples are then assessed for signs of poor sperm penetration. If there is a problem with either your sperm or mucus, this test should be able to identify which, as the donor sperm and mucus used have already been proven to function normally.

♂ Further investigations for the man

There are a series of additional tests that can be conducted on semen to assess its potential. These are generally only conducted in specialized clinics.

Sperm antibody testing

In some cases, antibodies may be found in the semen. This may also occur when a man has undergone vasectomy reversal or other surgery. Antibodies are not usually harmful, but they may have implications regarding further treatment.

Antibodies cause the body to recognize the sperm as invaders. Thus, they will attack the sperm and impair their function. A series of laboratory tests on sperm can be conducted to assess the presence and implications of sperm antibodies.

Women may also have antisperm antibodies, though uncommon, acting in the same way to impair the function of their partners' sperm. These may be present in the woman's mucus or blood and can be identified from mucus and blood samples.

Testicular exploration

If further investigations of sperm production and function are contemplated, these will usually involve referral to another special-ist, either an endocrinologist (a specialist in hormones and hormone-producing glands) or a urologist (a surgical specialist in the male genito-urinary tract).

There are a number of ways in which a specialist may want to investigate the testicles for signs of a blockage or a varicocele. A varicocele is a varicose vein around the testicles, although experts have disputed whether or not varicoceles are responsible for poor sperm quality.

Vasography

In the event that sperm *are* being produced but not found in the ejaculate, there is an X-ray procedure that can, in the same way as a hysterosalpingogram, reveal whether or not there is a blockage in the vas deferens, the tube conveying sperm to the penis.

Radio-opaque dye is introduced into the vas deferens, under general anaesthetic, and X-rays are taken to establish if there is a blockage.

Doctors may also confirm the presence of varicoceles using the Doppler effect or thermography. These methods are similar to ultrasound and can detect the heat generated in the area or the increased blood flow.

Exploratory surgery

In some indications, surgeons will operate to identify and, if possible, rectify any factors causing impaired sperm production. These indications are outlined in the next chapter.

Such operations are generally performed under general anaesthetic and may take a variety of forms, depending on the indications. If surgery is suggested, your doctor will explain the nature of the surgery and its implications beforehand.

The most common procedure is a small, exploratory operation, performed under general anaesthetic, which involves opening the scrotal sac to visualize the testicles, epididymis (where sperm are collected) and vas deferens (the tubes through which sperm travel to the penis). If a problem is discovered that is easily rectified, the surgeon may correct it at the same time. If indicated, testicular biopsy and vasography will be performed at the same time as the initial exploratory operation.

It is important to ask questions about why the surgeon feels it is necessary to operate and what it is hoped this will achieve. You should ask also how long you can expect to be in hospital and how much time you will need to take off from work. In general you will be in hospital for a day or two and should be able to return to work a day or so later, depending on the extent of the surgery.

Testicular biopsy

A testicular biopsy may be suggested when there is a complete absence of any sperm whatsoever or when there are very few, but the testicles are of normal size and hormone tests are normal.

It is a relatively simple procedure, during which a small sample of tissue is collected from the testicles for microscopic examination. This test is designed to show whether normal sperm are being produced that are not being expelled during ejaculation.

Urine sample

In a small number of men, the mechanism responsible for pumping sperm to the end of the penis acts in reverse. This is known as retrograde ejaculation. The sperm are pumped into the bladder, where they mix with the urine. A sample of urine taken after intercourse or ejaculation will demonstrate the presence of sperm.

♀ ♂ Summary

When investigations of both partners are complete, the doctors will arrive at a diagnosis. The time taken to reach this stage may be months or years. Your chances of arriving at a diagnosis quickly are improved if you attend one of the few clinics that have a specific interest in infertility.

You may have to keep pressing for further appointments and tests to identify the root cause of your problem, but appropriate treatment cannot begin until such a diagnosis has been reached. If appointments are booked to discuss results of previous tests, don't be afraid to telephone ahead to confirm that the doctor will have those results with him when you arrive. Particularly if you have experienced them not having come in in time before.

Keep a note of any results you have been given before so that you have them to hand. You may even find it helpful to keep a diary of your medical experience. Many couples find this quite helpful as it is entirely possible that you will meet new doctors at each appointment who want to go over your medical history each time. If you get this far in your quest to have a family, you are already becoming an expert on the subject!

4

Diagnosis, treatment, and outcome

Introduction

In this chapter, the possible diagnoses are described, along with first-line treatments that might be suggested for each diagnosis. 'Assisted conception' treatments are covered separately in the next chapter.

Not all doctors will prescribe the same treatment for any given condition, and there can often be disagreement between doctors about the usefulness of some procedures. Much of the information included in this chapter falls within the guidelines laid down for practioners in 1992 by the Fertility Committee of The Royal College of Obstetricians and Gynaecologists. Nonetheless, patients may still find themselves offered treatment that the Fertility Committee felt was inappropriate or of no value.

The most comprehensive research conducted into the causes, treatment, and outcome of subfertility was published by the specialist team at the University of Bristol under Professor Michael Hull, in 1985. The information and diagrams in this chapter are largely derived from this study of over 700 couples. This research is based on a sufficiently large and geographically defined group of patients to be considered representative of the population as a whole.

♀ ♂ *Counselling*

Before treatment begins, and often before a diagnosis is reached, clinicians have found counselling to be of great benefit to both partners. Counselling is a rather general term that, in this case, covers the need for you and your partner to explore your concerns about your subfertility, your investigations and what they might reveal, and any subsequent treatment.

Most specialist clinics have one or more members of staff whose role is specifically to help you talk through your fears and feelings, individually and as a couple. This person can also explain what treatment involves and help you cope with the implications of the diagnosis.

This person is not judging you or assessing your fitness as potential parents. The main aims of counselling are to reduce the stress of subfertility, to ensure you have all the information about your treatment and its possible implications that you require, and to provide support through what may be a very difficult time.

While a large number of subfertile men and women can be helped to conceive in time, a small number will have to accept that it will not be possible for them to have a child of their own. Another group of men and women will have to consider the prospect that the only way they may be able to experience parenthood is through the donation of eggs or sperm from someone else. The implications of this for both partners and any child born as a result of treatment are far-reaching. Some couples, as a result of this, and with the help of sympathetic counselling, find that they do not wish to proceed any further with treatment or investigation.

Counselling will help you cope with these difficult issues. Many patients and doctors also believe that effective counselling helps to reduce the stress of treatment, particularly assisted conception treatments, and this may improve the chances of ultimate success. Counselling is an important element of your clinical care – take full advantage of it.

♀ ♂ Diagnosis

The diagnosis will fall into one or more of the following categories:

- ovulatory failure
- tubal damage
- endometriosis
- mucus defect or dysfunction
- coital failure
- sperm defects or dysfunction and other male infertility
- unexplained infertility and other causes.

The most common causes of subfertility have been found to be ovulatory failure, sperm dysfunction, and unexplained infertility – these causes accounting for more than two-thirds of all subfertile couples (see Figure 4).

Once doctors have reached a diagnosis, a course of action will be suggested. You will want to know what your chances of achieving a pregnancy will be before you decide whether or not you wish to

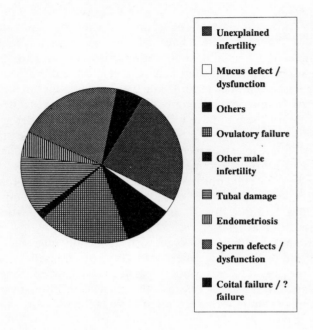

- Unexplained infertility
- Mucus defect / dysfunction
- Others
- Ovulatory failure
- Other male infertility
- Tubal damage
- Endometriosis
- Sperm defects / dysfunction
- Coital failure / ? failure

Figure 4. *The causes of subfertility.*

proceed with treatment. Just because treatment is available, does not mean that you have to have it or that it is your only option.

Treatment for subfertility can be lengthy, painful, expensive, stressful, and, in some cases, unsuccessful. For you to make an informed decision about how far you and your partner are prepared to go, you must have as much information as you can acquire about the general success of specific treatments in treating your diagnosed condition.

You can make the decision to stop treatment at any stage. With many conditions there is always a possibility that you may become pregnant without any treatment at all.

The outcome of various treatments, particularly assisted reproductive techniques, are subject to several variable factors, not least being the expertise of the doctors at the clinic. Using the general information given in this chapter you will need to get as much specific information from your doctor regarding your circumstances and the doctor's considered view before you decide whether or not to proceed with treatment. Bear in mind, also, that invasive surgical procedures and some drug therapies carry a small degree of risk of complications, some of which may be severe.

♀ Ovulatory failure

Ovulatory failure means that, for some reason, an egg is not being released from the ovary each month. The diagnosis may indicate that no eggs are being released at all or that the frequency of ovulation is severely reduced, impairing considerably the opportunities for conception. Even when a clear diagnosis of ovulatory failure is reached, partners' sperm function should still be confirmed before any treatment commences.

Conditions which give rise to ovulatory failure are:

- hormone deficiencies
- ovaries that are resistant to the body's hormone signals
- absent, damaged or diseased ovaries

Ovulatory failure is often characterized by absent, scanty, or irregular periods.

Absent or irregular periods

Absent or irregular periods mean that ovulation is also absent or irregular. The medical term for absent periods is amenorrhoea, and the term oligomenorrhoea (an abbreviated term for an even longer one) is used to describe infrequent periods. Amenorrhoea can further be categorized as primary or secondary. Women who have primary amenorrhoea have *never* had spontaneous periods, and women with secondary amenorrhoea have an established pattern of periods that suddenly stops. There are hormone treatments available to deal with these conditions, and the prospects of achieving a satisfactory outcome following treatment are generally good.

In the complete absence of periods where low body weight is considered to be a factor, methods of increasing body weight are essential before drug treatment commences.

If oral medication is unable to induce ovulation and regulate the cycle, other hormone therapies can be administered by injection. Such drugs usually cause the ovaries to generate more than one egg each month, so a multiple pregnancy may result.

The drugs most commonly prescribed to restore ovulation are clomiphene, in tablet form, human menopausal gonadotrophins, (hMG), and analogues of the human hormones FSH and LH, which are administered as injections. Some treatments are also administered by a slow pump injection, which mimics the pulses of hormone that the body releases naturally.

Clomiphene Clomiphene citrate, or Clomid, is widely used as a first-line treatment to induce ovulation. As a 50 mg tablet taken for five days early in the cycle, it has been found to be very effective in restoring ovulation. Usually the dose is repeated each cycle for several months and the results are monitored. The dose may be increased to two tablets, or 100 mg, per day for five days if required. Treatment with clomiphene alone can be very effective, inducing ovulation in about 70 per cent of women, and pregnancy in about a third of patients.

There are some mild side-effects reported with clomiphene. These include alterations to cervical mucus, making it more difficult for sperms to penetrate, and this may be the reason that more women do not conceive following restoration of ovulation with clomiphene. Other side-effects may include hot flushes, vaginal dryness, abdominal bloating, skin rash, nausea, dizziness, and depression. There is also a slightly increased risk of a multiple pregnancy.

Treatment with clomiphene is unlikely to be continued longer than six months without further investigations if pregnancy does not follow successful ovulation.

Clomiphene therapy may be combined with injections of hCG or hMG, but it is important that the results are monitored by the doctors throughout the cycle to confirm that ovulation is occurring and also to check the number of follicles that are developing in order to avoid the risk of a high order multiple pregnancy.

Other drugs that may be given to induce ovulation include cyclofenil, tamoxifen, and mesterolone. These are administered in a similar way to clomiphene and have a similar action.

Human menopausal gonadotrophin (hMG) hMG is widely used in assisted conception techniques, but can also be used to induce ovulation if other treatments have been unsuccessful. This hormone, known as either Pergonal or Humegon, is derived from human sources, the urine of post-menopausal women, which has been specially prepared and purified to isolate the two hormones, FSH and

LH. It is given as an intramuscular injection, into the deep muscle of the buttock, thigh, or arm.

These hormones exert a direct effect on the ovaries, causing them to produce several follicles and, subsequently, a number of eggs will ripen during the cycle. As this can lead to a greater risk of both a multiple pregnancy and ovarian hyperstimulation syndrome (see page 88) the use of hMG should always be monitored through ultrasound scans and hormone assessments, to establish the size and number of follicles developing in the ovaries.

If more than three follicles are found to be developing, great care should be taken to avoid the possibility of a multiple pregnancy. This may mean avoiding intercourse during the treatment cycle and waiting until a later cycle when the dose of hMG can be modified.

Full information regarding the administration of hMG can be found in Chapter 5, Assisted conception.

FSH is obtained by further purifying hMG to remove the LH. Although requiring an injection, it need only be introduced sub-cutaneously – that is, just under the skin – which is both easier and less painful than an intramuscular injection. While this preparation, Metrodin H.P., is more expensive than the combined preparation of hMG, the manufacturers claim that better results are achieved, but some specialists feel that apart from the greater ease of administration it is not any better.

It is likely that doctors will only try FSH alone when other treatments have been unsuccessful.

Luteinizing hormone releasing hormone (LHRH) is a hormone produced in the brain in an area known as the hypothalamus, which stimulates the pituitary gland to release FSH and LH. This hormone is also known as gonadotrophin releasing hormone (GnRH). The release of this hormone has been found to occur in tiny pulses, regularly, every hour or so.

In a small group of patients who do not respond to clomiphene therapy, the introduction of LHRH using a pump that mimics the natural rhythm of the pulses has been found to be very effective in restoring ovulation. This is sometimes referred to as pulsatile LHRH therapy.

The pump, which is carried around at all times, is attached to a syringe that contains a preparation of LHRH. The syringe is connected to a small needle inserted under the skin of the upper arm. Administration of LHRH with the pump is continued throughout the cycle, which is monitored with ultrasound scans to confirm that ovulation takes place.

Although the pump may feel cumbersome at first, most women find that they are able to continue with their normal daily work and activities without much inconvenience. There are few side-effects and less risk of ovarian hyperstimulation syndrome and multiple pregnancy than with hMG treatment.

When this treatment is given to women whose hormone problem is diagnosed as being hypogonadotrophic hypogonadism, the results are extremely good, with a pregnancy rate of around 90 per cent after 6 months' continuous use of the pump. The results in women diagnosed as having polycystic ovarian syndrome (see page 63) are less promising, at around 50 per cent after 6 months. This treatment has been found to be less effective when the woman is overweight. Pulsatile LHRH therapy is not effective for women experiencing premature menopause.

LHRH analogues A series of drugs known as LHRH or GnRH analogues has become available over recent years. These drugs, the most common being buserelin, are similar in chemical structure to naturally occurring LHRH, but have been slightly modified to alter their effects.

Although initially these analogues stimulate the pituitary gland to produce FSH and LH, after a few days of administration, the pituitary gland stops responding to both the drug and the body's own natural stimulus to produce these hormones. This effectively switches off FSH and LH production, which has a dual benefit. It prevents oversecretion of either of these hormones, which may be the causative factor in subfertility in some women, and it allows doctors to control, accurately, the amount of hormone available by subsequently introducing FSH.

Administering these analogues is complicated by the fact that it is not possible to take them orally as they would be destroyed by digestion, so they must be given either as an injection, an implant, or a spray inhaled through the nose. When LHRH analogues are used in conjunction with hMG it may be necessary to increase the amount of hMG given to achieve satisfactory stimulation; this increases the cost of treatment as both are expensive.

The administration of this combination is very common in IVF and GIFT treatment and further information about these can be found in Chapter 5, Assisted conception.

Monitoring treatment Whichever treatment programme is pre-scribed, it is reasonable to expect that its effects are monitored over the following months to ensure that it is working. If you have been following a prescribed treatment for more than a few months without success, ensure that you make another appointment at the clinic. Do not keep taking medication indefinitely unless you have been specifically advised to by the clinic doctor.

Some women have quite strong reservations about taking so many drugs when they feel they are not actually ill. Most of the hormone drugs described are derived from human or animal hormone sources, so they can be considered to be relatively close to the body's own. There is more concern about the LHRH analogues.

If you have any queries or worries regarding drugs prescribed for you, particularly those chemical analogues not derived from human or animal sources, express these to your doctor. Not all drugs that are newly available have a product licence for their use in ovulation induction and ovarian stimulation, and, while it is important that their usefulness be established, it is also important that full con-sideration is given to any possible long-term side-effects, which may not manifest themselves immediately.

New drugs are constantly being tested and assessed for their usefulness in assisted reproductive techniques and, at some stage, they must undergo trials involving patients. Your clinic doctor may invite you to be part of a research project using new treatment programmes or drug therapies. You have the right to decline to be involved if you feel you would prefer not to, without prejudice to any subsequent treatment. Make sure you satisfy yourselves fully about the nature of any research proposed, its potential usefulness, and its potential risks before agreeing to take part.

If you should experience any untoward side-effects, particularly pain or shortness of breath, while taking medication or following a course of medication, you should notify your clinic doctor or GP straight away.

One of the recognized side-effects of hormones used in the management of infertility is multiple pregnancy. It is important that doctors monitor the effectiveness of these drugs to avoid the risk of a high order pregnancy, such as quads, quins, or even sextuplets! A multiple pregnancy can be hazardous to both mother and babies, and the joy of parenthood can be seriously impaired when you and your partner are physically and mentally exhausted by having to meet the needs of three or more babies.

Doctors can visualize the number of eggs maturing in the ovary by means of ultrasound. In the event that too many are likely to be released together, doctors will advise you to use contraceptive protection until the following month, when the drug level can be moderated.

Hyperprolactinaemia

Amenorrhoea can be caused by oversecretion of the hormone prolactin, which is produced by the pituitary gland. One drug found to be effective in treating hyperprolactinaemia (that is, raised levels of prolactin) is bromocriptine. This is administered in tablet form. There may be some slight side-effects, such as nausea, and vomiting when taken without food. Bromocriptine is normally effective within a few weeks, restoring ovulation and a normal chance of conceiving.

Very occasionally, hyperprolactinaemia may be caused by a benign (harmless) tumour of the pituitary gland. This can usually be identified with an X-ray or CT scan of the skull (CT stands for Computerised Tomography scan, a diagnostic technique that allows doctors to visualize the structure of an organ by producing images of sections, or 'slices', of the organ). This is not a cancerous tumour and responds well to bromocriptine. In the event that the tumour does not respond to bromocriptine, which occurs in about 10 per cent of cases, doctors may suggest either surgery or radiotherapy to remove the tumour and restore prolactin levels to normal. Bromocriptine is usually stopped once pregnancy is established.

Modern surgery for prolactinomas (as these tumours are known) is relatively straightforward, leaving no visible scar and requiring around a week in hospital. Radiotherapy may be used to reduce the size of a tumour following surgery. Further X-rays or CT scans can confirm that the tumour has responded to treatment and blood tests can verify that prolactin levels are normal.

Abdominal surgery to restore ovulation Prior to the availability of the hormone treatments previously described, doctors would resort to surgery in an effort to restore ovulation. Ovarian wedge resection was performed, and is still occasionally suggested, particularly in the treatment of polycystic ovarian syndrome.

In a wedge resection, a small slice of the ovaries was removed during a major surgical abdominal operation. This was found to restore ovulation in over half the patients. The risk of further complications, such as bleeding and the formation of scar tissue

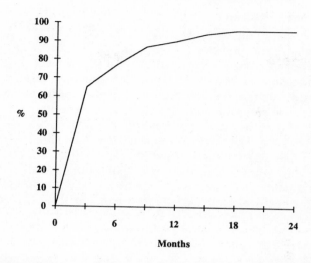

Figure 5. *Cumulative conception rates in couples with amenorrhoea only.*

around the ovaries and Fallopian tubes, meant that there was a real possibility that the tubes might become blocked, so this procedure is rarely performed today.

Premature menopause

Sometimes referred to as premature ovarian failure, this can occur at any age and there is no effective treatment that can restore the function of the ovaries, although, very occasionally, they may recover spontaneously.

In the event that your ovaries are absent or completely unable to respond to drug therapy, the option now exists for egg donation. By this means eggs are obtained from other women who have agreed to be donors. You would receive hormone replacement therapy at the same time, to maintain the uterus in a state of readiness for implantation.

Donated eggs are fertilized with your partner's sperm for replacement, as an embryo, into your womb. This carries with it a slightly better success rate than IVF, providing your partner's sperm is adequate and no other reason exists that might make it difficult to sustain a pregnancy. Ova donation is considered in more detail in Chapter 5, Assisted conception.

The outcomes of treatments

Figure 5 shows the outcomes of all the treatments described for women with amenorrhoea who don't have a premature menopause. The vertical axis shows the percentage of women who achieve pregnancy and the horizontal axis shows the time taken in months. It can be seen from this that, after 6 months of treatment, nearly 75 per cent of women treated become pregnant, and, after 2 years, 96 per cent.

Figure 6 demonstrates the conception rate for women with oligomenorrhoea. Here over 50 per cent of women conceive after 6 months, while a plateau is reached at around 70 per cent after 18 months. This indicates that there is no point in persisting with the same treatment after this time, when it might be appropriate to conduct further investigations, alter the treatment, or stop treatment altogether.

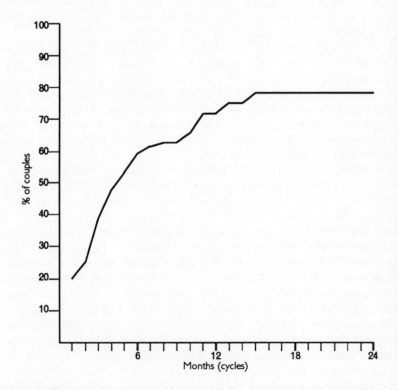

Figure 6. *The cumulative conception rates of women with oligomenorrhoea*

Polycystic ovarian syndrome

This is sometimes referred to as polycystic ovary disease. It usually becomes evident as a result of an ultrasound investigation or laparoscopy, and then it can be seen that the ovaries are enlarged and covered with small cysts. Women diagnosed as having polycystic ovarian syndrome may have erratic periods, unwanted body and facial hair, and greasy skin or acne, arising from oversecretion of the hormone testosterone. Excess weight may be part of the problem. The syndrome may cause ovulation to fail in some cases and this is why it causes subfertility, although many women are known to have polycystic ovaries and experience no symptoms whatsoever.

Doctors have discovered that excess weight may make the condition worse, and so are likely to prescribe an appropriate diet to start with. If test results reveal a hormone imbalance, either tamoxifen or clomiphene may be used to restore ovulation. If this fails, the hormone pump may be used or other forms of super-ovulation, as described earlier.

In the event that none of these treatments is effective, ovarian diathermy (a minor operation performed using a laparoscope) may be suggested.

Using either a laser or electrodiathermy equipment, small areas of the surface of each ovary are sealed by heat. This has been found to improve ovulation in some cases, although doctors tend to reserve its use for slim patients, as the procedure is more difficult to carry out for those women who are overweight.

♀ Tubal damage

This refers to damage to the Fallopian tubes, which may prevent sperm from meeting the egg. Fallopian tubes often become obstructed as a result of infection arising from, perhaps, appendicitis, peritonitis, previous abdominal surgery, gonorrhoea, or chlamydia. The damage may block the tubes or cause adhesions. Adhesions are sheets of fibrous repair tissue, which, during the process of recovery from infection or surgical intervention, may weld structures together or encapsulate the ovaries. Extensive adhesions may block the tubes, distort them or reduce their mobility. Even very slight damage can cause a marked degree of subfertility.

Damage to one tube is not necessarily an indication for further treatment. Many women with only one tube manage to achieve pregnancy with time, even if they have only one ovary working on the opposite side. It is quite possible for an egg released from the right ovary to be collected by the fimbria of the left Fallopian tube. It is only when there is blockage or severe damage to *both* tubes that treatment is necessary.

There are two main approaches to treatment of tubal damage: tubal surgery and IVF, which requires special facilities not widely available so you may need to be referred to another clinic. Tubal surgery, though, can often be performed at district level, providing there is an experienced surgeon.

Tubal surgery may be the first choice where the tubal damage is slight, giving a pregnancy rate one year after surgery of up to 60 per cent. Women over 35 and those who have had previous tubal surgery are less likely to succeed than those under 35 where surgery is performed for the first time. If tubal damage is severe, the subsequent pregnancy rate falls quite markedly. If, after surgery, pregnancy does not occur within 12–24 months, IVF will then be the remaining option. Where tubal damage is severe, IVF may be the only viable option.

The Fallopian tubes are delicate and about the same size as the lead in a pencil. To operate successfully on a patient with moderate tubal damage, a surgical microscope is usually used to enable the surgeon to visualize the tubes more accurately. During the operation, the surgeon delicately removes areas of adhesion or damage and attempts to restore the ovaries and tubes to their correct positions. This is a major operation; it is performed under general anaesthetic and may last up to several hours, depending on the severity of the damage. A hospital stay of around seven to ten days is required and it may be six weeks before you can go back to work.

The success of this operation depends on a number of factors. The site of the damage to the tubes may have a considerable bearing on the outcome. Up to 45 per cent of patients may be successful if the blockage occurs at the point where the tubes meet the uterus. If the damage is in the region of the fimbrial ends of the tubes, closest to the ovaries, the outcome is much less satisfactory, closer to 10–30 per cent. Another factor governing the outcome of tubal surgery is the degree of experience and expertise of the surgeon.

Contemplating major surgery for subfertility is a difficult matter. Most surgery is performed because a patient is sick or in pain. This is not so for the subfertile woman who, apart from the mental pain of her infertility, is young, fit, and healthy.

Ectopic pregnancy

There is an additional risk that, following surgery, the adhesions will return and, in the event of moderate to severe damage involving the Fallopian tubes, there is a risk of ectopic pregnancy. This occurs when a developing foetus lodges in the tube instead of progressing to the womb. This occurs in about 10–15 per cent of pregnancies following tubal surgery. This is a dangerous condition that may necessitate further major surgery to remove the foetus and, often, the affected Fallopian tube, too.

If you have tubal surgery, it is important to be aware of the signs and symptoms of an ectopic pregnancy. If you miss a period you will obviously be very aware of the likelihood of pregnancy, so it is a good idea to notify the clinic anyway. An ultrasound scan performed 14 days or so after your missed period should be able to confirm the presence of a uterine pregnancy or an ectopic one.

If the foetus lodges in the tube, it will continue to grow and manifest all the early signs of a normal pregnancy. In time, however, the tube will become distended, which will lead to pain, and, eventually, the tube will rupture and start to bleed. It is not usually possible to save the foetus if this happens. Ectopic pregnancy may be particularly dangerous for the woman, causing considerable blood loss and, possibly, collapse.

Doctors will usually investigate as a matter of urgency, starting with a laparoscopy to identify the cause of the bleeding. If an ectopic pregnancy is confirmed, the doctor will usually proceed to perform a laparotomy. This is an operation in which an incision is made in the lower abdomen to allow access to the tube. On occasions, it is possible for the foetus to be removed without removing the tube, depending on the site and degree of damage, but most often the tube and the foetus are removed. If the site is close to the ovary it may sometimes be necessary for the corresponding ovary to be removed as well.

The most common signs of ectopic pregnancy are pain in the abdomen and vaginal bleeding. You may also feel faint. These are also the symptoms of a threatened miscarriage, so when you consult your doctor, *make sure he or she knows you have had previous tubal surgery* as this increases the likelihood of ectopic pregnancy considerably. Another more obvious sign of ectopic pregnancy is pain in the tip of the shoulder. This is known as referred pain as it arises in response to internal bleeding in the abdomen.

The impact of an ectopic pregnancy is often quite considerable. Not only have you lost the baby you so wished for, but you may have lost one Fallopian tube as well. Unfortunately, because of the damage any surgical intervention can cause, there remains a risk that there may be a further ectopic pregnancy in the future in the remaining tube.

♀ Endometriosis

This is a condition in which some of the cells lining the womb spread along the tubes to cover other adjacent organs. These cells bleed, in the same way as does the endometrium in the womb during menstruation, which can lead to scarring and blood-filled cysts. This causes pain and can lead to marked subfertility. Some women who have endometriosis experience painful periods, heavy periods, or pain on intercourse, while others may experience no symptoms whatsoever.

Many women suffering from this condition can conceive and bear a family with no difficulty, but it is thought that endometriosis is more likely to be found in women who have delayed childbearing. Up to 40 per cent of subfertile women may be found to have endometriosis, although it may not be the primary cause of their subfertility.

The management of this disease is very much dependent on the degree of damage it has caused. Doctors categorize the disease by the degree of severity, ranging from minor to moderate and severe. Figure 7 shows the pregnancy rates for untreated patients with varying severities of endometriosis in comparison with normal pregnancy rates. It can be seen that severe endometriosis, particularly affecting the ovaries, has a significantly poorer outlook in this respect than does minor to moderate endometriosis.

If the condition is mild and giving rise to no real symptoms, such as painful or heavy periods and pain on intercourse, and has only been diagnosed following a laparoscopy, despite the fact that it is comforting to think that you have finally uncovered the root of your problem, it is possible that doctors will not treat the endometriosis at all. As mentioned earlier, many women conceive when they have endometriosis, so it may not be a primary causative factor of subfertility. Some of the experts believe that such patients should be treated as though they had unexplained subfertility.

The doctor has several options for treating endometriosis. The first proposal might be hormone treatment to halt menstruation for

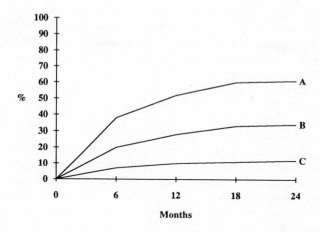

Figure 7. *The conception rate in couples with unexplained subfertility (A), endometriosis not involving ovaries (B), and endometriosis involving ovaries (C) without treatment.*

several months in order to allow the damage to repair itself. If extensive scar tissue and cysts have been discovered within the pelvis, your doctor may advise surgery to remove areas of disease and adhesions. This might involve a major operation, but, in some cases, it can be done through a laparoscope using a laser. There is a view among experts that, unless the disease is causing marked symptoms, there is no value in undertaking this treatment.

A combination of surgery and hormone treatment may be appropriate in severe cases, but, if this proves unsuccessful, IVF remains the last available option. Endometriosis is one condition where it is particularly difficult to get the experts to agree on which course of action is most appropriate. We have, therefore, outlined some of the most common treatments in use, for your information, along with the comments of the experts.

Minor endometriosis may be treated with hormone drug therapy. It has been proved that the symptoms of endometriosis subside when menstruation ceases, either through pregnancy or menopause. This can be artificially induced with a number of drugs currently available.

One drug commonly used is danazol, which induces a temporary menopause. Unfortunately, such drugs have a contraceptive effect and so will only be used in the short term (six to nine months), after which, if treatment is successful, menstruation will resume and the disease will be no longer suppressed. During the treatment, the endometriosis regresses and will, hopefully, remain suppressed when treatment ends. Around one-third of women will have a recurrence over the following four years and around one-third of women with mild endometriosis will conceive following this treatment. However, research shows that an equal proportion would have conceived without any treatment.

Side-effects from the drugs used are likely to be those associated with the menopause – hot flushes, weight gain, and vaginal dryness. They may also include nausea, slight hair loss, and acne. All these effects will disappear in time, once the drugs are stopped. The major disadvantage is the fact that the drugs act as a contraceptive and so pregnancy cannot be achieved until the treatment ceases. This is particularly stressful for older women, who feel that they are already running out of time.

The verdict of the Fertility Committee of the Royal College of Obstetricians and Gynaecologists on this treatment was: 'Most certainly the prescription of ineffective medication that is contraceptive in a group of infertile women is unjustified.'

In severe cases, surgery is performed to try to remove areas of the disease, any adhesions that may have formed, and to free any organs that may have become attached. This may take the form of a major, microsurgical operation (such as that described in the section on tubal damage) or it may be possible to remove much of the disease using a laser during laparoscopy. This is much less invasive than a major abdominal operation and has the additional advantage of a lower likelihood of post-operative adhesions forming. This facility, however, tends only to be found in specialist fertility clinics.

Whatever treatment is suggested, the outcome can be extremely variable, depending on the severity of the disease and other factors, such as partner's sperm. With management, between 10 and 60 per cent of endometriosis sufferers will become pregnant after one to three years.

Where all other treatments have failed, or where the severity of the disease is considered to be unamenable to treatment, IVF remains the only option. However, some specialists believe that women with mild to moderate endometriosis who have been infertile more than two or three years should be offered IVF.

♀ *Mucus defect or dysfunction*

In incidences where your partner's sperm fail to penetrate your mucus, the most common cause is likely to be sperm dysfunction. If, however, on sperm/mucus crossover interaction testing your partner's sperm is found to penetrate *donor* mucus successfully, the indications are that it is your mucus that is resistant. This is often termed mucus 'hostility' and is relatively rare, being responsible for only 3 per cent of all subfertility.

Mucus hostility may arise as the result of an infection, such as thrush, or perhaps a hidden infection that is symptomless. This can usually be detected by taking a high vaginal swab and testing it. Antibiotics or antifungal agents may be prescribed to eliminate the infection.

Anti-sperm antibodies may be found in the mucus, which could destroy the sperm. These may result from previous infection and should subside once the infection has been treated. Antibiotic treatment may be offered to both partners to prevent one partner from passing the infection back to the other during intercourse.

Intra-uterine insemination (IUI)

In the event that no sign of infection or antibodies is found, the treatment suggested for mucus hostility may be intra-uterine insemination (IUI). This involves the preparation of a sperm sample from your partner, which is introduced directly into the uterus at the time of ovulation. This is repeated every month or every other month. This treatment might also be suggested for unexplained infertility and some cases of poor sperm quality.

Because sperm are introduced directly into the uterus, an ordinary semen sample cannot be used as it is not sterile, so the semen sample is prepared and washed before it is introduced through a fine plastic tube, called a catheter, through the neck of the cervix.

On its own, this treatment is unlikely to be much more effective than ordinary intercourse. To improve the chances of success, IUI is often combined with superovulation. Superovulation is a means of increasing the number of eggs available for fertilization during the treatment cycle (see page 56). Hormone drugs are given to the woman during the first part of her cycle, and her ovaries are monitored by means of blood or urine samples and abdominal ultrasound to check the number of eggs developing.

One of the disadvantages of this type of treatment is the possibility of a multiple pregnancy as there is always a risk that *all* the eggs produced might be fertilized. This is why it is so important that egg development is monitored and, in the event that more than three eggs are found to be developing, insemination should not take place.

This treatment offers a success rate of up to 30 per cent over 6 to 18 months. Such repetitive treatment places a considerable strain on a couple, and, after 12–18 months without success, further investigation may be required. If sperm quality is proven, IVF or GIFT treatment may be the next options.

♀ ♂ *Coital failure*

To achieve pregnancy, the penis must fully penetrate the vagina and deposit semen close to the cervix. If, for any reason, this is not occurring, or not occurring at the right time, then pregnancy will not follow.

There may be physical or psychological problems that prevent successful coitus. Where there are psychological difficulties, couples may be referred to a psychosexual counsellor before any further fertility treatment is considered.

In the event that a relationship has not been consummated, this may be as a result of vaginismus. This is a condition in which the muscles of the vagina involuntarily go into spasm whenever intercourse is attempted. If this has a psychological origin, it can usually be overcome by means of sensitive counselling and instruction in the use of vaginal dilators. If the reason is physical, it may arise from either painful endometriosis or vaginal infection, which can generally be treated successfully.

In some situations, intercourse is being practised in such a way that sperm are not allowed to remain in the vagina long enough to swim up through the cervix, perhaps because of withdrawal of the penis before or at the moment of ejaculation. This is easily overcome if the man keeps his penis inside the vagina until after he has ejaculated.

Some couples have been advised, wrongly, to 'save up' the sperm for the 'Right Day'. This is bad advice, however, as sperm quality is likely to decline considerably if there has been a long period of abstinence.

Bathing or using a douche immediately after intercourse may destroy sperm or wash them away and lubricating jellies should be avoided as these might also be harmful to sperm.

Failure to achieve an erection or to ejaculate will also result in coital failure. There may be a physical reason for this or a psychological one. The stress of being unable to achieve an erection is unlikely to diminish as the pressures of subfertility grow.

Premature ejaculation can usually be overcome with the help of careful counselling and instruction for both partners. Using manual stimulation, the woman can bring her partner close to ejaculation. By squeezing his penis just below the glans, before ejaculation can occur, the urge to ejaculate will be reduced. This manual stimulation and squeezing can be repeated until control is improved and intercourse attempted. This can generally be achieved within a few days.

Impotence, an inability to maintain an erection, may arise as a result of a number of known clinical conditions or may be caused by psychological problems. Appropriate medical help will be required for the underlying cause of impotence, but these problems can generally be overcome by artificial insemination with partner's sperm – usually referred to as artificial insemination by husband (AIH). The sperm are introduced by syringe into the vagina during the time of ovulation. It can be repeated over successive days if necessary. This is a relatively simple procedure that can be conducted at home. If it does not succeed over a period of six months, doctors may prefer to do the insemination in the clinic, using the partner's sperm, which they can prepare in such a way as to improve its performance. Further investigation may be merited if this is unsuccessful after 6–12 months.

If no other problem is identified, the chances of achieving pregnancy are good.

♂ Sperm defects or dysfunction

Sperm disorders are the single most common cause of subfertility, and remain one of the hardest to treat successfully.

Sperm defects can be divided into two categories: oligozoospermia (often referred to as oligospermia), and azoospermia. Oligospermia means a reduced output of sperm, and azoospermia means there is an absence of any sperm in the ejaculate.

In the event that a serious problem is discovered with successive sperm analyses, and there has been found to be no problem with your partner, your clinician has two options. It might be possible for you to undergo further investigation and treatment at the clinic you are attending, or another specialist clinic, or the doctor may feel that the only way in which you and your partner will be able to have a child is by insemination with sperm from a donor.

Following the considerable advances in the management of female infertility during the 1980s through assisted conception techniques, there has been a greater concentration on research into male factor infertility. Over recent years, new techniques have been developed to improve the chances of fertilization with poor-quality sperm. The method and outcome of treatment for sperm defects is very much dependent on the degree of defect, rather than on the total number of sperm.

Figure 8 shows the conception rates over 24 months for couples treated as a result of producing a negative post-coital test – that is, the sperm failed to survive mucus penetration. Two groups were

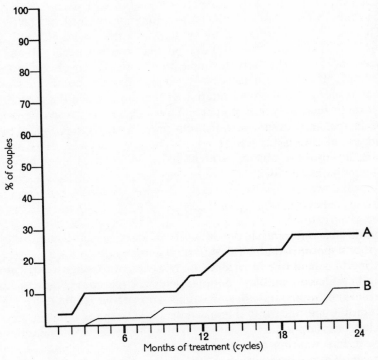

Figure 8. *The cumulative rates of conception in couples who receive treatment after a negative post-coital test: A = normal, B = oligospermia and failure to penetrate mucus*

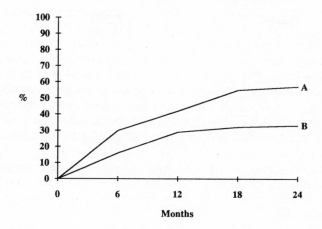

Figure 9. *Conception rates for previously subfertile couples where motile sperm densities are more (A) and less (B) than 4 million per ml. (without treatment) and the female is normal*

assessed: one in which the male partners had normal semen specimens, and one in which the specimens were oligospermic. The outlook for couples where the semen was oligospermic were poorer than that for those with normal sperm.

In research involving 286 couples who had previously been subfertile, where no disorder had been diagnosed in the female partner, conception rates over a period of 18 months, during which time no treatment was given, were measured. Figure 9 shows a considerable difference in outcome for two groups – one in which the partner's sperm had a motile density greater than 4 million sperms per millilitre and one in which the motile sperm density was lower than 4 millions per millilitre. Motile sperm are those sperm that are of normal appearance and function when viewed under the microscope.

If motile sperm density is greater than 4 millions per millilitre, the doctors' first approach might be to suggest more frequent inter-course, the wearing of boxer shorts, and, possibly, bathing the testicles in a cool bath, although the latter two suggestions have little clinical evidence to support their usefulness. From the research documented in Figure 9 it can be seen that, after 12 months, nearly half the couples achieved conception without further treatment. After 12 months or so without success, further treatment may be considered.

It is apparent from several clinical studies that as many as 30 per cent of men with suboptimal sperm quality will have a partner who also has a problem. It may be the case that slightly reduced fertility on the part of both partners may be a real contributory factor in their subfertility, meaning that their chances of success without treatment are considerably less than the norm of around 25 per cent. In this situation, many doctors will opt to treat the female partner to optimize her chances of becoming pregnant with the sperm as it stands.

Oligospermia

In those cases of oligospermia for which a cause can be found, the treatment varies according to the diagnosis:

Contact with toxic substances Environmental or occupational exposure to toxins, such as pesticides or drugs in manufacture, is usually quickly discovered and treatment obviously involves withdrawal from the toxic environment. The outcome is dependent on the length of time of exposure, but the outlook is generally good.

Other medication Drugs used in the treatment of ulcerative colitis and cancer may have a deleterious effect on sperm quality. It might be possible in the case of ulcerative colitis for the drugs to be altered to decrease the effect on the sperm.

Treatment for cancer – whether in the form of chemotherapy or irradiation – may cause irreversible damage to the testicles. For this reason, where possible, doctors treating the cancer will often arrange for the collection and frozen storage of the man's semen so that it can be retained for many years in the event that he may wish to try for a family at a later date. The semen can then be thawed and introduced into his partner by artificial insemination. Unfortunately, the outlook for such patients may be disappointing as there may be little time after diagnosis of cancer to collect sperm specimens before treatment commences and, because of the illness, the sperm quality may be poor.

Varicocele

This is a varicose vein around the top of the testicles. It is not fully understood why a varicocele may affect fertility, although it has been argued that the decreased blood flow through the vein may cause an increase in the temperature of the testicles, thus affecting sperm production.

Many fertile men have a varicocele and so it is not necessarily a cause of subfertility. To diagnose this condition, you stand upright and strain down or cough while the doctor feels the scrotum.

Treatment usually involves an operation to remove the varicocele, by tying off the abnormal veins through a small incision in the groin. This is performed under general anaesthetic and may require taking two to three days off work.

There is little clinical evidence to demonstrate that pregnancy rates are increased as a result of this operation, but this does not mean it is not a useful and sometimes effective treatment, particularly where sperm counts and motility are low and there is no other obvious explanation for subfertility.

Infection

Signs of infection may be apparent in a semen sample either through the presence of white cells or a reduction in sperm production and motility. The effect of previous infections, such as gonorrhoea, tuberculosis, and chlamydia, may cause blockage of tubes transporting sperm from the testicles.

Treatment for infection will depend on the pathogen found to be responsible. Appropriate, long-term antibiotic therapy may improve the semen quality sufficiently to restore fertility. In some cases, both partners will be treated to prevent the possibility of one partner reinfecting the other during intercourse.

Antisperm antibodies

Antisperm antibodies may be treated with high-dose steroids. These may suppress antibody levels, but they also carry some level of risk as steroid drugs also impair the body's natural defence mechanisms. Some success has also been achieved by direct intra-uterine insemination with prepared partner's semen – and quite good success has been achieved with IVF.

Morphological abnormalities

These are abnormalities in the appearance of the sperm. They are usually congenital – that is, something that one is born with, not something that develops in later life. In the event that all the sperm are abnormal, there may be nothing that can be offered in terms of treatment – except with some of the newer micromanipulation techniques (see p. 100).

Undescended testicles

If the testicles are late in descending into the scrotum, doctors will usually operate to rectify this when the child is still young to avoid subsequent subfertility. The effects on sperm function may be helped by hormone treatment, but, if the damage is considerable, this may be of little help.

Mumps orchitis

Mumps orchitis is not just mumps. It is when mumps involves inflammation of the testicles, and it occurs in around one-third of men who contract mumps after the age of 12. In one-third of these, the result is azoospermia. In others, sperm production may be reduced. The damage is caused at the time of infection, and there is little that can be done to reverse the effects of this damage.

Hormone deficiency

In the event of a very low sperm count, blood tests are conducted to assess the levels of two hormones: FSH and testosterone.

A high level of FSH indicates that the testicles are not capable of responding to the body's hormone signals. This is difficult to rectify and the prospects are poor. A normal FSH level accompanying azoospermia is indicative of a blockage. This is usually investigated further by surgery. If the blockage is easily rectified, the outlook is good – but in general the results are poor.

A low level of FSH may indicate the presence of a pituitary tumour. Further blood tests and X-rays may be performed to verify this. A pituitary tumour, which can occur in men and women, is *not* a cancerous growth. It can generally be treated by taking bromocriptine tablets, which will rectify the hormone imbalance and cause the tumour to shrink. The outlook as a result of this treatment is good.

Low levels of testosterone require treatment to overcome the symptoms, which include hair loss, lethargy, and impotence, but it is unlikely that sperm quality can be improved. Tamoxifen tablets may be given to regulate testosterone levels, but if an improvement is not detected within the first month of treatment, the outlook is unpromising. In the event that a rise *is* detected, treatment is likely to be continued for six months.

Azoospermia

Azoospermia refers to a total absence of sperm in the ejaculate. This may arise as a result of a number of causes.

Blockage If there are no sperm found in the semen sample, this might be due to a blockage, which is preventing the sperm produced from reaching ejaculation. In addition to restorative surgery, doctors have another treatment option. It is sometimes possible to collect sperm directly from the epididymis, where the sperm are manufactured. These sperm can then be introduced directly into your partner's uterus at the time of ovulation, or they can be collected in this way and then used as part of an assisted conception technique, such as GIFT or IVF, and introduced to the egg directly. If the sperm are normal, then the prospects are good.

Retrograde ejaculation In the event of retrograde ejaculation, sperm are pumped backwards into the bladder rather than forwards into the partner's vagina. It may be possible to collect sperm from a urine sample produced immediately after ejaculation. These sperm can then be specially cleaned and prepared for artificial insemination.

Primary testicular failure This is a complete failure of the testicles to produce any sperm at all. This may arise from a hormone deficiency or a failure of the testicles to respond to hormonal stimulation. This is relatively rare, accounting for less than 5 per cent of male subfertility.

If azoospermia arises from a hormone imbalance, it may be possible to regulate this with tablets or injections, which will stimulate the testicles into normal sperm production. It may, however, be difficult for doctors to understand *why* primary testicular failure has occurred. Then, if treatment is unsuccessful in overcoming the problem, the only remaining option is donor insemination.

Vasectomy

Some couples, once they have completed their families, feel sure that they want no more children, so they opt for vasectomy as a permanent and safe means of ensuring this. Vasectomy is a contraceptive procedure designed to prevent sperm from being ejaculated. The vas deferens is blocked on both sides during a minor surgical procedure.

Occasionally, though, some couples change their minds about

wanting more children or their circumstances change. In particular, following divorce, a vasectomized man may meet a new partner and they may decide they want a family together. In this event, vasectomy reversal is the only option other than donor insemination.

Surgery to rejoin the tied ends is usually the only method of reversing vasectomy. It is difficult to predict the outcome of reversal as, although the operation to restore the vas deferens is usually completely successful, antisperm antibodies often form following the vasectomy. In high concentrations, these antibodies will impair sperm performance and this is generally found to be untreatable. Functionally, around 80 per cent of men may have a successful repair of the vas deferens and about 60 per cent of their partners will conceive over a 2 year period.

Doctors used to think that the length of time that has elapsed since the vasectomy was performed might have a bearing on the success of vasectomy reversal, but this is not now felt to be the case.

A sperm sample is collected following the reversal operation to gauge its success. In the event that sperm quality is poor or no sperm are found, donor insemination is then the only option.

The outlook for men in whom sperm production is severely impaired is improving as doctors research to find ways of collecting even a very small number of sperm surgically from the epididymis of the testicles for direct introduction to their partner's egg. Epididymal sperm aspiration and donor insemination are covered in Chapter 5, Assisted conception.

♀ ♂ *Unexplained subfertility*

Unexplained subfertility is defined as a failure to conceive after one to two years of unprotected, regular intercourse when accurate investigations have revealed normal menstrual cycles, normal semen analyses and sperm/mucus penetration, and no detected abnormality after carrying out a laparoscopy.

As human fertility is naturally a rather inefficient process, quite a large number of couples will simply have been unlucky not to have become pregnant in this time, and, over the next year or two will find their luck will change. Research has shown that 80 per cent of couples who have been trying for up to 3 years became pregnant in the following 18 months, while this figure dropped to around 40 per cent if they had been trying for 3–5 years, and 30 per cent if they had been trying for longer than 5 years (see Figure 10).

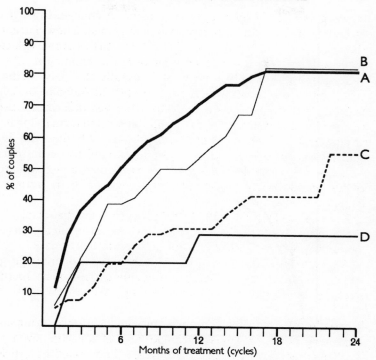

Figure 10. *Cumulative conception rates in couples with unexplained subfertility related to the duration of subfertility at the time of the first clinic appointment: A = 1–2 years' wait before treatment, B = 2–3 years, C = 3–5 years, D = 5 years and more*

It is important when arriving at a diagnosis of unexplained subfertility that the investigations are of the highest standard. There may well be an identifiable problem, but perhaps only a specialist clinic is equipped to identify it. After more than 3 years of unexplained subfertility, the chances of conception become greatly reduced, at around 30 per cent. Those women who are older have an even lower prospect of conception. Figure 11 compares the cumulative pregnancy rate for women who are under 25, 25–29 years, 30–34 years, and over 35. There is a slightly better outlook for those with secondary subfertility.

There is no obvious treatment programme for unexplained subfertility, but doctors may suggest intra-uterine insemination, GIFT or IVF. IVF provides an additional diagnostic opportunity over other

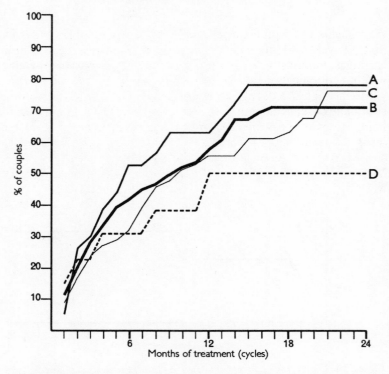

Figure 11. *The cumulative rates of conception following treatment of couples with unexplained subfertility related to the age of the woman: line A denotes under 25, line B 25–29, line C 30–34, line D 35 and over.*

treatments as it allows doctors to see whether or not follicle development and egg production are normal, and whether or not fertilization is occurring. The success rate for IVF in unexplained subfertility is good, at around 20–25 per cent per cycle. If repeated attempts at IVF or GIFT are unsuccessful, the only remaining options are to try using donor sperm or donor eggs.

It has not been proved that stress or some other psychological factor plays a part in unexplained subfertility, but more and more doctors are exploring this area by means of drama therapy, psycho-therapy, and counselling.

♀ ♂ *Miscarriage*

As many as 1 in 5 pregnancies ends in miscarriage, often within the first 12 weeks of pregnancy. Some women suffer repeated miscarriages, but most will, in time, go on to have a full-term pregnancy without complications.

Miscarriage is a deeply distressing experience, causing profound shock and bereavement in both partners and family. It is not possible here to cover the subject of miscarriage effectively. For further information and support both CHILD and ISSUE can help, as well as The Miscarriage Association (for their addresses, see pages 144–5). You might also like to read *Talking about Miscarriage* by Sarah Murphy.

5

Assisted conception

Introduction

By the time assisted conception is considered to be appropriate treatment for you and your partner, it is likely that you have already spent some considerable time, energy, and money trying to become pregnant. If you have not already been referred to a specialist or tertiary referral centre, this should now happen. The next chapter, Choosing a clinic, will deal with how to find the best clinic for your needs, taking into account the fact that you may have to pay for all or some of your treatment, while this chapter deals with what assisted conception actually involves. It is important to read all the information in this chapter even if you know which treatment programme is likely to be appropriate for you as much of the information is pertinent to all forms of assisted conception.

The permutations on the ways and means of becoming parents made possible by assisted conception techniques are considerable. It is now possible for a woman to bear a child who is neither genetically hers, nor her partner's. It is also possible for another woman to carry a child on behalf of an infertile couple, where both sperm and egg come from the originating couple. There are several more variations on this theme. It is crucial, then, as this involves the lives of children, that these unprecedented developments are not subject to abuse. Furthermore, it is important to establish, in the eyes of the law, just who the legal parents are.

♀ ♂ *The law and assisted conception*

Unlike almost any other form of medicine, assisted conception involving the use of human gametes (eggs and sperm) and embryos is governed by an act of Parliament, The Human Fertilisation and Embryology Act, passed in 1990.

This arose as a result of the increasing public concern about the possible uses and abuses of human reproductive material that could occur, particularly regarding eggs, sperm, and embryos. It was felt that there should be a code of practice governing its conduct and an overseeing body to ensure that the guidelines laid down were followed, in the interests of doctors, patients, and children born as a result of assisted conception.

The Human Fertilisation and Embryology Authority (HFEA) was duly set up in 1991 to license practising clinics, without which they are not authorized to undertake IVF, human embryo research, or treatment involving donated eggs or sperm. These licences are subject to annual review, and if they are withheld or withdrawn it is unlawful for the specified treatments to be carried out.

The Act further states that patients must have 'been given a suitable opportunity to receive proper counselling about the implications of taking the proposed steps, and have been provided with such relevant information as is proper'. This is particularly important. The treatments described in this chapter can place an enormous amount of stress on the men and women receiving them. Clinics have a legal obligation to provide information and counselling about the implications of treatment as a part of the treatment offered. There should be no surprises about what is involved in the treatment or what may be the outcome.

The Act also places a responsibility on doctors to satisfy themselves that any child born as a result of regulated treatment, or who might be affected by the birth of such a child, is taken into account: 'A woman shall not be provided with treatment services unless account has been taken of the welfare of any child who may be born as a result of the treatment (including the need of that child for a father) and of any other child who may be affected by the birth.'

This is a difficult issue to interpret as, on the one hand, couples do not want to feel that they are being judged as to their suitability as prospective parents, while on the other, no one wants to feel that insufficient consideration has been given to the future needs of children who might result from treatment.

In practice, doctors need to satisfy themselves that you have a good relationship with your partner and that you have given consideration to how you might tackle issues such as disclosure of the origins of the child. Doctors and counsellors will want to explore your attitudes to children born as a result of donated eggs or sperm. You might also like to consider the attitudes of extended family members to such a child, whether you choose to disclose its origins or not.

The part of the sentence quoted regarding the need of the child for a father does not necessarily mean that single women and lesbian couples cannot be offered treatment, but it does force the doctor to take this need into account when deciding whether or not to provide treatment.

The Act also makes provision for the collection of data relating to the provision and outcome of regulated treatments. This data is stored by the HFEA and remains completely confidential.

Although *any* treatment for subfertility might be regarded as assisted conception, the majority of treatment is designed to help you conceive on your own. The term 'assisted conception', as it implies, refers to treatment where doctors *assist* with the conception process itself.

The main forms of assisted conception are:

- gamete intra-Fallopian transfer (GIFT) (not a treatment requiring a licence from the HFEA)
- in vitro fertilization (IVF)
- donor insemination (DI).

These three treatment methods are usually, though not always, performed in conjunction with ovarian stimulation. This maximizes the opportunities for achieving pregnancy with each treatment cycle.

♀ Ovarian stimulation

There are several ways of administering the hormones required to control and stimulate the ovaries to produce more than the single egg normally produced each month. These may include tablets, injections, nasal inhalations, or small slow-release pellets or implants inserted under the skin.

Your clinic doctor will decide on the best drug programme for you, which may start some months or weeks before the treatment cycle. In preparation, some clinicians have found that taking the Pill for a few months beforehand is helpful, to regulate the cycle before introducing the ovarian stimulation hormones.

One group of drugs commonly used to increase control of the cycle is gonadotrophin-releasing analogues, which include buserelin, nafarelin, decapeptyl, and goserelin. These are given as a 'sniffer', that is, to be inhaled, or as an injection, or an implant. These are frequently used in the weeks before treatment commences as they are known to suppress the hormones that govern the development of the eggs, which allows doctors to control the cycle with much greater accuracy and so reduce the distressing possibility that a treatment cycle may have to be abandoned if the eggs are released too soon.

The drugs most commonly used to stimulate the ovaries are very similar to human hormones. They are, clomiphene, given in tablet form, and human menopausal gonadotrophins (hMG) – Pergonal, Humegon, or Metrodin HP – given as injections, or a combination of both (these are discussed more fully on page 56). Clomiphene may also be used in conjunction with LMG.

Usually your clinic doctor will outline your proposed drug programme when you are accepted for treatment, but is unlikely to be able to prescribe your drugs for you on the NHS.

The cost of drugs

If you *are* receiving this treatment on the NHS, you will already know that there is little or no funding for assisted conception, so it is unlikely that there will be provision in the hospital budget for these very expensive drugs. This will mean that you will have to persuade your GP to prescribe them for you, but if the doctor won't or can't do this, you will have to buy them with a private prescription.

It is over issues like this that many infertile couples really despair. Not only is this treatment rarely available within the NHS, but, on top of the cost of private treatment, many are expected to meet the costs of expensive drugs as well. This is one of the reasons it is important to establish a good relationship with your GP – his or her support could be very valuable at this time.

The drugs listed are not commonly stocked in all chemists and it is advisable that you obtain your drugs before your treatment cycle commences. This will reduce any unwarranted stress. If, however, your treatment cycle is cancelled, it is not possible to return the drugs to the pharmacy once they have been dispensed. Once you know you have all your drugs ready, it is also important to organize for them to be administered.

Administering ovarian stimulation drugs

Pergonal, Humegon, and Metrodin HP are presented in ampoules, small glass phials containing white powder. Included in each pack is another, smaller glass phial containing a clear fluid, marked sterile diluent. These are given together as an injection.

It is usual for the drug regimen to require two or more ampoules each day. These will be administered together, generally at about the same time of day, including weekends.

It may be possible to receive your injections at the clinic, if you live nearby and they have staff on duty every day. If you live further away, your GP may arrange for the practice nurse to give you your injections during the week and the duty nurse to do so at the weekends.

If your GP is unwilling or unable to help you, you may have to make your own arrangements. A friend living nearby who is a doctor or a nurse might help.

Many couples have overcome this difficulty by learning to do it themselves. It is possible for a woman to learn to inject herself, or to have her partner inject her. This is a lot easier than it sounds and reduces the stress considerably. You can then have your injections in your own home and you will both feel more involved in your own treatment.

There are now self-injection kits available with some of the drugs, but otherwise you will need to obtain a supply of needles and syringes. It may be a good idea to draw up the drug using a different needle from the one you inject yourself with as you may find that they become rather blunt. Always discard needles, syringes, and glass phials carefully after use, and never reuse a syringe or needle. Your clinic may be able to give you a special sharps container for disposing of your injection material safely.

If you want to inject yourself, your clinic nurse will be able to teach you how to do your injections. It is best to do the first few in the presence of the nurse in case you get into any difficulties, after which you will feel more confident. Whoever administers the injection, though, it is useful to know how to draw up the drug, as you may find your GP or nurse is unfamiliar with it.

Although each packet contains both the drug and the diluent, you do not need to use more than one phial of diluent if you need more than one phial of drug.

The phials are designed to open by snapping off the top cleanly at the ring around the neck. Some packs include a simple device to enable you to remove the top of the ampoule easily. A sterile syringe is attached to a needle. This is used to draw up the diluent first, and this is then squirted into the powder, which immediately dissolves. This liquid is then drawn up into the syringe. If further ampoules are prescribed, the fluid in the syringe is then squirted into the remaining phials and drawn up in the same way.

Up to five phials of powder can be diluted with one phial of diluent. The remaining phials of diluent can be discarded. Do not allow a nurse or doctor who is unfamiliar with the drug to use one phial of diluent with each prescribed phial of powder as this could be a very large and very painful injection.

The injection is administered either into the muscle bulk, usually the buttock or thigh in the case of Humegon and Pergonal, or just under the skin (subcutaneously). More drugs are being designed for subcutaneous administration to make it easier for patients to administer themselves. If you *are* doing this yourselves, make sure that the clinic nurse shows you exactly where to inject.

The sniffer

Unlike the other drugs discussed, buserelin and nafavelin are designed to switch off hormone production by acting directly on the pituitary gland, which controls all hormone activity. This allows for greater management of the subsequent treatment cycle, but may mean that a greater dose of the other drugs is required to achieve the desired stimulation.

These drugs, known as LHRH analogues are administered in an unusual way: by sniffing it into each nostril. You may be asked to start sniffing on the first day of your period or around day 21 of the cycle, immediately before treatment commences. Some clinics will ask you to sniff every four hours. Depending on your daily routine, you will establish the best timing for you. Many find that the least disruptive schedule is to sniff at 11.00 a.m., 3.00 p.m., 7.00 p.m., 11.00 p.m., 3.00 a.m., and 7.00 a.m. Some clinics will allow you to omit the 3.00 a.m. sniff while others use more recently available drugs, which only require a twice-daily sniff.

A similar drug is also available in injection form, and as a slow-release pellet, which is placed under the skin.

Once your doctor is satisfied that your hormone levels have been suppressed so that it is possible to control ovarian stimulation directly, you will be instructed to begin your daily injections, which may be given in conjunction with the sniffer, or tablets, or both.

Side-effects and risks

There are several minor side-effects that patients experience after using the drugs described. These are similar to the effects of the menopause – hot flushes, irritability, sleeplessness, and headaches. Once the other drugs have started to be used and the ovulatory cycle resumes, these symptoms will pass.

The objective of ovarian stimulation, sometimes called 'super-ovulation', is to recruit more than three ripe eggs. On average, up to 10 follicles will develop, but for 20 or 30 to develop is not unknown! Each fluid-filled follicle is easily visualized on the ultrasound screen, and the scanner can measure the diameter of each follicle on progressive days to assess their development.

It does not necessarily follow that each follicle will contain an egg and so ongoing hormone tests (using blood or urine) may be performed to measure levels of oestrogen, a hormone produced by developing eggs.

Ideally, all the main follicles will be of a similar size. On some occasions, one follicle may appear to dominate, by being larger than the others. If this happens, it may mean that this egg will ripen first. If this follicle erupts, releasing the egg, a hormone will then be released that will suppress the other smaller follicles, which means that they will not reach maturity. Doctors may elect to deliberately 'lose' this follicle to allow them to recruit the remainder.

It is not always possible to tailor superovulation drugs accurately for all women, so treatment programmes may have to be amended in order to achieve the best outcome. This may mean that a treatment cycle does not proceed if the response has been insufficient. This is sometimes referred to as 'abandoning' a cycle and you may feel pretty abandoned yourself if this happens! Generally, if a cycle has to be postponed, your doctor will suggest a brief break to allow your system to return to normal and prescribe a different drug programme for your next attempt.

There is a risk associated with superovulation known as 'ovarian hyperstimulation syndrome'. This can cause cysts to develop on the ovaries and fluid to collect in the abdomen. This may mean that the treatment cycle has to be abandoned and the superovulation programme for the next cycle altered. In very few cases, ovarian hyperstimulation syndrome may be severe, requiring urgent treatment in hospital. *Symptoms such as nausea, vomiting, abdominal pain, and shortness of breath must always be reported to the clinic without delay.*

If ovarian hyperstimulation syndrome is diagnosed at or following egg collection for IVF or GIFT patients, doctors may elect to freeze any embryos produced from eggs collected and replace them at a later date when the condition has regressed. This is only possible at clinics with full laboratory facilities or those with access to such facilities.

Once the scan indicates that a number of eggs are approaching maturity, ovulation is artificially induced as this minimizes the risk of the follicles releasing their eggs before the team is ready to collect them. To do this, an injection of another hormone, human chorionic gonadotrophin (hCG) is given, which can be predicted to induce ovulation 34–36 hours later.

Egg collection or insemination is frequently scheduled to be carried out in the morning, so it is not unusual to be told to have your hCG injection at an awkward hour. If your operation is scheduled for 9.00 a.m., for example, your injection will be 34 hours before, at 11.00 p.m. This is a very good argument for learning to inject yourself! You might be able to arrange, through your GP, to have this injection at the local hospital if you can't do it yourself.

♀ ♂ *Gamete intra-Fallopian transfer (GIFT)*

The word 'gamete' is used to describe the two cells – the sperm and the egg – that combine together to form the embryo. The GIFT technique involves the collection of one or more eggs, which are mixed with sperm, then replaced in the Fallopian tubes. It is a lengthy and stressful procedure, carrying a success rate in the region of 25 per cent per treatment cycle.

GIFT treatment is slightly more accessible than IVF as it is easier to set up and clinics are not obliged to abide by the guidelines laid down by the Human Fertilisation and Embryology Act. High-tech laboratory facilities are not a necessary requirement, although some laboratory facilities are required to assess eggs collected and prepare the sperm so more clinics are able to provide the service. For this reason, GIFT may also be a less expensive option than IVF.

GIFT treatment is indicated for:

- some cases of endometriosis
- unexplained subfertility of more than two to three years' duration.

Not all doctors agree on the indications for GIFT treatment, and some experts feel that IVF is more useful as it gives evidence that fertilization is taking place. Some licensed clinics will suggest a preliminary IVF cycle in cases of unexplained subfertility or reduced sperm quality as a way of assessing fertilizing ability, followed by subsequent attempts at GIFT, once fertility is proven, if the first IVF cycle does not result in pregnancy.

GIFT, unfortunately, is not a regulated procedure, which means it can be performed in a centre that does not have a licence. While this might mean that treatment may be accessible nearer to home or at less expense, it also means that unlicensed practitioners do not have to meet the high standards required by the HFEA.

This treatment is only rarely available, free of charge, within the

NHS. Generally, if your doctor feels that this is the appropriate treatment for you and you do not want to go on to a long waiting list, you may have to consider seeking private treatment. You might consider entering your names on the nearest NHS GIFT waiting list and seek private treatment in the meantime.

♀ *What is involved?*

After preliminary investigations and procedures have been completed, you should have the opportunity to discuss at length with a member of staff at the clinic what treatment involves, how long it is likely to take, and what the possible outcomes may be. Good clinics will have informative, clear, written instructions for you to take away. A consent form will be completed before treatment commences.

Once you have been accepted for treatment, you will be asked to contact the clinic on the first day of your next period. This is the start of a treatment cycle and so should be counted as day 1. The start of your period is when you first see red blood.

Some clinics may advise you that, if your period begins *before* midnight on a Tuesday, for example, you must count the Tuesday as day 1; if your period begins any time *after* midnight, you must count the Wednesday as day 1. This is variable from clinic to clinic – some may set, say, 5.00 p.m. as the break-point.

The clinic will normally request that you attend for an ultrasound scan on day 1 or 2. This is called a baseline scan, which allows doctors to assess your ovaries to ensure that no cysts are present and to take measurements of ovaries and uterus. Cysts on the ovaries can occur at any time and they tend to be transient. A cyst is a fluid-filled sac.

Occasionally, a cyst may respond to the hormone treatment given to encourage more eggs to grow in each ovary. If this happens, the cyst, too, might grow and become uncomfortable for you. For this reason, your doctor may advise you to miss this cycle and return next month, when the cyst is likely to have subsided.

If the scanning doctor is satisfied with the first scan, then you will be advised to start your medication. The dose and frequency of medication varies from clinic to clinic and patient to patient.

Scans are performed over the ensuing days to measure the development of the eggs. In conjunction with blood or urine analysis, the scans will indicate that the eggs are nearing maturity and, once they are ready, the hCG injection is given and egg collection is arranged to take place 34 hours later.

Egg collection This procedure is usually performed under general anaesthetic by laparoscopy. The whole procedure takes about 40 minutes and you will usually be allowed home about 4–5 hours later. If you are given a general anaesthetic, you will be unconscious during the whole procedure.

Your clinic will advise you not to eat or drink before your operation. They may need to do a final ultrasound check before operating to ensure that you have not ovulated prematurely. Your partner must, of course, accompany you, so that he can provide the semen for inseminating the eggs, unless frozen or donor sperm is to be used.

During the operation, the surgeon is able to see the ovaries and Fallopian tubes through a long fibreoptic tube, which is inserted through a small incision near the navel. Using special equipment, the surgeon will collect each ripe egg from each ovary. These will be passed to the embryologist, who will store each egg in special media in an incubator. Once all the accessible eggs have been collected, the embryologist will study them under a microscope to decide which are the best.

Up to three of the best eggs will be mixed with a sample of washed and processed sperm. These eggs will be replaced inside the Fallopian tubes on both sides.

All the main follicles will be emptied in the search for eggs as it is important that no eggs are left to ovulate later. This is because up to three eggs are replaced, all of which have the potential to develop into a foetus. Any additional eggs left to mature may also add to the risk of a multiple pregnancy.

SPARE EGGS In the event that more than three eggs are collected, there are a number of ways of dealing with them, providing the clinic is licensed.

If the clinic has full IVF laboratory facilities, any spare eggs can be inseminated with your partner's sperm. This is a very useful diagnostic test as it will indicate whether or not your eggs will successfully fertilize with your partner's sperm. If your spare eggs are inseminated with your partner's sperm but do not fertilize, however, this is not necessarily an indication that fertilization is impossible, because the best eggs will always be replaced during the operation, so that those available for insemination may have been of poorer quality.

If embryos *do* result, your clinic may have facilities to freeze these spare embryos for you to try to achieve a pregnancy in the future. The HFEA guidelines permit clinics to inseminate eggs they cannot freeze for one purpose only, which is to establish whether or not fertilization is occurring. After this, all spare eggs that cannot be inseminated and subsequently frozen must be discarded. Unfortunately, it is not yet possible to freeze unfertilized eggs.

You may also be asked whether or not you might consider donating any spare eggs or embryos, particularly when a large number are collected, either for use in research or for donation to other infertile couples who are unable to produce their own eggs or sperm.

You and your partner need plenty of time to consider the implications of donating spare eggs or embryos, and you should not feel under any pressure to do so. Talk it through with your partner and clinic counsellors at length before you make your decision, which should be made well in advance of your egg collection so that you don't feel rushed.

Research on human eggs and embryos is very important because it allows doctors to improve infertility treatments, to develop new drugs, and to understand more about human fertilization. If you do feel that, say, if more than ten eggs are collected you would like to donate those not required for your treatment for research or for other couples, you will be given a detailed consent form explaining what you have agreed to, which you will both have to sign. Even if you sign this consent form, you can change your mind at any time, providing the eggs or embryos have not already been used.

These are very important issues, so it is vital that the staff of the clinic discuss all the possible outcomes with you both *before* you start treatment. You must also decide, before treatment, how many eggs you would like to have replaced. It is recommended that no more than three should be replaced. This is to minimize the risk of a multiple pregnancy. You can ask for fewer eggs to be replaced once you have discussed your chances of success with your doctor.

You and your partner may feel that a multiple pregnancy would be acceptable, even desirable. Although by far the majority of patients who undergo IVF or GIFT treatment successfully actually have a single pregnancy, the rate of twins or more being born following GIFT when more than one egg is replaced is about ten times greater than would be expected in the general population.

Having waited many years for your family, it would be a shame to have so many children at one time that you are unable to enjoy one because you are exhausted meeting the needs of several! Couples who have had triplets, quads, and more have found that they need round-the-clock help for the first few years, and that a high order multiple pregnancy can be very expensive as well as exhausting.

Even if only three eggs are replaced, the potential exists for one of the eggs to split into two, as happens naturally with twins. There have been several reported cases of quads resulting from GIFT where only three eggs were replaced. For this reason, where sperm quality is good and the woman is under 30, doctors may suggest restricting the number of eggs replaced to 2, particularly if this is your first treatment cycle.

It is very important, before treatment commences, that the clinic treating you counsels you both fully about the physical and ethical implications of GIFT treatment, after which you should both sign a consent form.

GIFT is a demanding process, taking a lot of time, particularly in the later stages of ovarian stimulation. You may be required to attend the clinic day after day. Apart from your injections, you will have frequent blood tests and perhaps urine tests. In general, doctors will want to try GIFT treatment once or twice, but, in the event of unsuccessful treatment, IVF might be suggested as the next course of action, as more diagnostic information regarding fertilization could be available using this method.

Variations of GIFT

This procedure is sometimes called T-SET, which stands for Tubal Sperm Egg Transfer, but, essentially, it is the same procedure as that just described.

GIFT egg collection may be performed by ultrasound rather than using a laparoscope (this is described more fully in the next section on IVF). If eggs are collected by ultrasound, the patient does not necessarily need a general anaesthetic, although some form of sedation is given, but the eggs may have to be replaced using a laparoscope to see the Fallopian tubes. It is also now possible for the eggs and sperm to be placed in the Fallopian tubes using ultrasound-guided replacement through the uterus.

Some clinics will also try GIFT on a natural cycle – that is, without superovulation. While this reduces the costs and stress considerably, the chances of success are reduced as there is only going to be a single egg and the risk of spontaneous ovulation occurring before egg collection is slightly higher.

ZIFT is another procedure that is similar to GIFT, but which can only be practised at a licensed centre. Here, eggs collected are fertilized and replaced at what is called the 'pronuclei stage', which occurs the day after egg collection. When the egg and sperm fuse together during fertilization, a single cell is formed with two pronuclei – one from the egg, one from the sperm. This is the first sign that fertilization has taken place. This cell, or zygote, is then replaced in the Fallopian tube, hence the name zygote intra-Fallopian transfer – ZIFT. As fertilization is thought to occur naturally in the Fallopian tube, this procedure may be slightly more successful than IVF as it more closely imitates the natural reproductive process. Another advantage of this procedure over GIFT is that fertilization is known to have taken place before the cell is replaced.

DIPI, or DIPSI, means 'direct intra-peritoneal injection, or sperm injection' (the peritoneum is the membrane that lines the abdominal cavity, covering the abdominal organs).

In this procedure, prepared sperm are introduced directly into the abdomen, thereby meeting the egg without having to pass through the vagina, cervix, uterus, and Fallopian tubes. This might be particularly helpful where sperm motility is reduced.

This treatment works on the principle that the sperm will meet the egg as it erupts from the ovary, and this will then be picked up by the fimbrial ends of the Fallopian tubes. If superovulation is used in conjunction with DIPSI, doctors will need to ensure that no more than three eggs are likely to be produced to avoid the risk of a high order multiple pregnancy. This usually means giving clomiphene tablets alone. This treatment is not suitable for women who have damaged tubes.

POST is yet another variation, meaning 'peritoneal oocyte sperm deposit'. This involves egg collection, usually by ultrasound, and the subsequent deposit of eggs and sperm back into the abdominal cavity near the Fallopian tubes, where, it is hoped, they will be picked up by the Fallopian tubes. This, again, requires that the tubes be undamaged.

It is possible to perform GIFT using donated eggs, donated sperm, or, indeed, both. If eggs are donated, obviously the egg collection operation is unnecessary and the donated eggs are mixed with the partner's or donor sperm and introduced into the Fallopian tubes during laparoscopy, after appropriate hormone preparation.

The outcome of GIFT

After the replacement, the most difficult and stressful part begins:

the wait. To know whether or not treatment has been successful, you must either return to the clinic 12–14 days after your operation for a pregnancy test or have a test done at home if you live some distance from the clinic, if your period hasn't started. The last few days before your pregnancy test are extremely trying – every time you visit the toilet you will be checking for signs of a period.

The chances of achieving a pregnancy vary according to a number of factors. Overall, throughout the country, GIFT clinics are achieving a success rate of between 20 and 25 per cent per cycle commenced. This means that 20–25 per cent of women who begin a treatment cycle will become pregnant as a result.

The factors governing success are the degree of expertise of the clinic staff, the age of the woman, and the cause of the subfertility. If there has only been a small, borderline problem with perhaps sperm function or ovulation, the combination of superovulation and direct introduction of sperm may be all that is needed. Chances of success are increased if you have become pregnant by your partner before, are under 35, or your partner's sperm quality is good.

If you become pregnant, the risk of miscarriage is slightly higher than in the general population. The increased possibility of a multiple pregnancy may contribute to this, though it has been known for one foetus to miscarry while its twin goes on to full term.

There is also about a 5 per cent risk of ectopic pregnancy. Your clinic will be watching for this if you are found to be pregnant. Occasionally, however, pregnancy is not obvious when it is lodged in the Fallopian tube, so, if you feel any unusual pain a few weeks after your operation, make sure you let the clinic know. Patients have described the pain of ectopic pregnancy as a dull abdominal pain accompanied by a sharp pain in the shoulder or chest that is similar to wind pain.

Assisted conception and your work

If you are working, you may not have told your colleagues and employer that you are seeking treatment to help you become pregnant. Few employers are sympathetic about treatment that takes you away from work repeatedly, and sometimes at short notice, particularly if the result might be a worker who ends up taking maternity leave!

It might not be possible to book holiday leave either, because doctors cannot predict exactly what day treatment will start and when egg collection is likely to be. If you book annual leave and treatment is postponed, abandoned, or prolonged, you may find that you cannot easily cancel or alter it.

While some clinics will try to be flexible about scanning times to fit in with your work, most are busy and tend to have the day organized around scanning sessions and egg collections, offering little leeway for juggling appointments. If you live a long way from the clinic, it might be even more difficult for you to work around your appointments. You will certainly need at least one day off work for the operation for egg collection, and possibly a day or so after, until you feel fully recovered.

You will have to decide whether or not to tell your employer about your treatment. It is very possible that your employer will know someone who has been through something similar and they may be more sympathetic than you think. Alternatively, they may make a difficult time even more problematic if they prove unhelpful. You need to minimize the stress in your everyday life so you can cope with the considerable burden treatment will put on you. You owe it to yourself to give yourself the best chance of success.

♀ ♂ *In vitro fertilization (IVF)*

The name of this technique stems from the fact that fertilization takes place in a glass container. Thus, it is sometimes known as the 'test tube baby' technique.

IVF is primarily indicated for women with blocked or damaged Fallopian tubes, when tubal surgery has been unsuccessful or is inadvisable. It is also frequently attempted where a wide variety of other problems have been diagnosed, including endometriosis, male factor subfertility, unexplained infertility, cervical insufficiency, and ovarian dysfunction. IVF may also be suggested after GIFT treatment has failed.

IVF success rates have improved considerably since the birth of the first IVF baby in 1978. The pregnancy rate consistently achieved in some of the more successful clinics is now approaching 25 per cent for women under 40 with partners who have acceptable sperm function. This is equal to, and in some cases better than, the chances of achieving a pregnancy naturally when there is no fertility problem.

The procedure for IVF is exactly the same as for GIFT in terms of ovarian stimulation. IVF differs at the point of egg collection.

♀ *Egg collection*

There are a variety of ways in which eggs can be collected. Unlike GIFT, where doctors need to visualize the ends of each Fallopian tube to replace the eggs and sperm, in IVF, the eggs are fertilized in the laboratory.

It is not always necessary to have eggs collected under a general anaesthetic, through the laparoscope. Some clinics will collect eggs while the patient is sedated, under ultrasound direction. This means that drugs are used that render the patient sleepy and relaxed. Painkillers are usually given at the same time. This method of collection saves time and money, meaning that the patient can go home around four hours after the procedure.

By using an ultrasound probe, the doctor can locate each follicle. He or she can then direct a needle through the bladder or the vagina into each follicle to reach the eggs. Despite the sedation and painkillers, this is quite an uncomfortable procedure, lasting between 45 and 60 minutes.

Whether the eggs are collected by laparoscope or ultrasound, with the patient sedated or anaesthetized, will depend on the clinic. Some will only have one method of collection, while others may offer all.

Once the eggs have been collected, they are taken to the laboratory where they will be inseminated with washed and processed sperm, from either your partner or, if appropriate, a donor.

The eggs are then placed in a special incubator designed to mimic the conditions found inside the body. The eggs will not be disturbed until the embryologist checks the following day to see whether or not fertilization has occurred. The day after egg collection, you will be contacted by the clinic who will tell you how many eggs have fertilized. If the eggs have fertilized, you will return, usually the following day – that is, two days after egg collection – for embryo transfer.

Embryo transfer

The guidelines under which clinics operate dictate that they may not return more than three embryos. This is to minimize the risk of a high order multiple pregnancy.

Embryo transfer is a relatively simple procedure, taking about ten minutes. The doctor places a small catheter into the neck of the cervix (a catheter is a small, flexible tube attached to a syringe). The embryos are drawn into the catheter in the laboratory and then deposited inside the womb. This is rarely a painful procedure, although occasionally a small instrument has to be used to steady the cervix and this can result in a small, sharp pain being felt. Occasionally, embryo transfer can be done under general anaesthetic.

Opinions vary about whether or not it is advisable for the patient to lie still for an hour or so following embryo transfer. Your clinic will have a policy about this, but there is no evidence to suggest that there is any greater chance of a pregnancy if you do rest.

Some clinics will also prescribe further hormones to provide endometrial support – that is, support for the lining of the womb to help it sustian the embryo(s). This may be in the form of injections, tablets, or the use of pessaries around the time of embryo transfer, particularly where buserelin has been used. Opinion is varied about the usefulness of this.

Following embryo transfer, it is always difficult to know what to do next. Most clinics advise taking things easy for the following day or so, then doing everything you would normally do afterwards, with perhaps the obvious exceptions of no heavy lifting, horse riding, and other strenuous pursuits.

There really is no right or wrong thing to do after embryo transfer, but perhaps the best advice is to occupy yourself fully with something that will help to take your mind off wondering whether or not treatment has been successful.

♀ ♂ *Variations of IVF*

IVF can be performed using either donated sperm or donated eggs. Where sperm are donated, the process is exactly the same as that laid out on page 102 regarding donor insemination. Following egg collection, the selected donor sperm are thawed and prepared before being introduced to the eggs in the normal way. Embryo transfer follows successful fertilization.

Cryopreservation This is the freezing and storage of sperm or embryos. For quite a while now, doctors have been able to freeze and store sperm for long periods of time, which can then be thawed for use at any time. However, techniques for successfully freezing and thawing human eggs have not yet been perfected, but it is now possible to freeze a *fertilized* egg or embryo.

This ability is particularly useful for IVF and GIFT patients who produce spare eggs. These can be inseminated and if they successfully fertilize, they can be frozen so that the couple can have another chance of achieving a pregnancy without the need for another treatment cycle first. This has another advantage in that the embryo can be replaced in a cycle where no superovulatory drugs have been used to distort the natural cycle, although hormone replacement therapy may be given to emulate a natural cycle.

The success rate for frozen embryos is around 11 per cent live birth rate per frozen embryo transfer, but there is no guarantee that all embryos frozen will survive the thawing process. Currently around 75 per cent of frozen embryos will thaw successfully.

It is particularly important for couples who have spare, frozen embryos to decide what they would want to happen to the embryos if their circumstances were to change. This is particularly important in the event of the death of one or both partners, or separation or divorce. This should be considered before a treatment cycle commences, and your decision should be noted in the consent form that both partners must sign.

Transport IVF and IVC Two modifications to IVF have been developed to make IVF more affordable and more accessible to a greater number of couples.

One of the greatest expenses of IVF is the laboratory facility, which is primarily used to examine, store, and fertilize the eggs and sperm. The key feature of the laboratory is the incubator, an expensive piece of equipment that is set up to mimic the conditions found in the uterus. A fully commissioned and staffed laboratory facility is usually only found in central clinics, which may mean couples need to travel long distances to receive treatment. This is particularly stressful and expensive when it involves repeated journeys for scans and blood tests.

Many district hospitals have the facilities to monitor superovulation and collect eggs, but they don't have the laboratory facilities necessary to fertilize the eggs. 'Intra-vaginal culture' (IVC) is one way around this problem. Eggs collected are mixed with partner's sperm in a specially designed tube, which is placed inside the vagina of the woman and held in place with a diaphragm or cap. The vagina itself acts as an incubator, keeping the eggs at the right temperature and the woman feels little or no discomfort.

After 24–48 hours, the tube is removed and the contents examined for signs of fertilization. If fertilization has occurred, up to three embryos are returned to the uterus. This is particularly helpful for women with blocked tubes.

Transport IVF also involves the initial monitoring and egg collection being performed at the local district hospital but, in this case, laboratory facilities are provided at a central clinic.

The woman's partner produces his semen sample on the day of egg collection, at the central clinic, where he is given a portable incubator that he then takes to the hospital where the egg collection is taking place. After the eggs have been collected, they are placed in the incubator, which he then returns to the central clinic. The eggs are then inseminated at the central clinic, where, if fertilization has occurred, embryo transfer will be performed two days later.

This process can be quite stressful for the male partner, but may save on the cost of treatment.

♂ *Micromanipulation of sperm* Developments in IVF techniques have led to improvements in the management of male factor subfertility. The most innovative techniques involve using a single sperm or a very small number of sperm, which are introduced to the egg in a variety of ways. This is of particular value where the motility of the sperm is poor or where only a very small number of sperm are available.

Doctors in Nottingham have developed a technique known as Computer Image Sperm Selection (CISS), which they hope will help them select the best sperm from a sample for use in these techniques.

Where there is a history of blockage or where vasectomy reversal has been unsuccessful, specialists are developing ways of collecting a few sperm directly from the testicles. Microepididymal sperm aspiration (MESA) and percutaneous sperm aspiration (PESA) are still in their infancy, but, already, pregnancies have been confirmed where the sperm collected are introduced directly into the egg. MESA involves an open surgical operation while PESA allows doctors to extract the sperm through a special needle, introduced through the skin under local anaesthetic.

The egg has a tough protein shell – known as the 'zona pellucida' – that a sperm has to penetrate to fertilize the egg. Sperm whose motility is poor or whose structure does not permit penetration can be introduced directly to the egg by artificially bypassing the zona pellucida.

There are several methods by which this can be achieved, although they are all still the subject of much research and ongoing refinement. One method, known as sub-zonal insemination (SUZI), involves a small number of prepared sperm being introduced into the space between the egg and the surrounding membrane.

Intracytoplasmic sperm injection (ICSI) works on the same principle as SUZI, although, in this case, the sperm is introduced directly into the cytoplasm (the inner cellular structure of the egg).

Some clinics are working on finding ways of opening the zona pellucida artificially, by either drilling a hole using an acidic culture medium – known as zona drilling – or by inserting a tiny glass needle into the zona, making a small hole, allowing sperm an easier passage to the egg – known as partial zona drilling. These techniques require some forward progression of sperm.

At present, such treatment is very expensive and success rates are poor. Figures published in 1992 by the HFEA estimated that up to 60 per cent of patients reached embryo transfer, 7 per cent of these established a pregnancy, and, of these, around 25 per cent subsequently miscarried. In time, these results are likely to improve, but, in the meantime, couples will have to consider very carefully whether or not they feel that an expenditure in excess of thousands of pounds is worth it for a treatment whose success rate is lower than 5 per cent. There are currently seven clinics researching this type of treatment in the UK.

This treatment is currently available, under licence, from a limited number of clinics. A list of these clinics is available from the HFEA.

♀ The outcome of IVF

If, 12 days after embryo transfer, your period has not occurred, you will have a pregnancy test. Some clinics favour a sensitive blood test, which needs to be done by a doctor, while others prefer a urine test, which you can use at home, to detect biochemical pregnancy, although this may not lead to a live birth.

The success rate for IVF is improving all the time. Good clinics can now expect a live birth rate of around 25 per cent per treatment cycle, where sperm quality is good and the woman's age is under 40. This success rate is equal to the natural success rate for any normal fertile couple. If the treatment were not so costly and complex, IVF could be helpful for a large number of subfertile couples.

The number of times IVF is attempted may depend on a number of factors. Some NHS clinics may only offer up to three attempts, after which patients must find another clinic if they wish to try again. Some private clinics will happily treat couples as many times as they are prepared to pay for the treatment, providing previous treatment cycle results have been favourable. Other couples find that NHS treatment is not available to them, perhaps on grounds of age, previous children, or location, and they simply cannot afford the cost of private treatment.

If treatment *is* available, providing all goes well during an IVF cycle and doctors can see no reason for you not being successful in time, it might be worth considering three attempts at IVF. Some couples find just one attempt so stressful they could not repeat it, while others return again and again (this aspect is discussed in more detail in Chapter 8, What next?)

It may be that you go to several different clinics over a period of years for treatment. You may find small variations in the way some aspects of treatment are handled. By and large a clinic follows a particular programme because it is what they have found to be most effective. It does not necessarily indicate that any one course of action may be right while another is wrong.

♀ ♂ *Donor insemination (DI), or artificial insemination by donor (AID)*

The indications for DI are:

- poor-quality or low numbers of sperm (oligospermia)
- complete absence of sperm (azoospermia)
- any genetic disorder that makes it inadvisable for your partner to father a child
- rhesus incompatibility, where previous pregnancies have resulted in stillbirth or severely affected babies
- male disability
- vasectomy or failed vasectomy reversal.

Genetic disorders are not necessarily associated with subfertility, but in a situation where you are known to carry the gene of a disease such as Huntington's Chorea or haemophilia, using donor sperm will eliminate the risk of passing the gene on to your child.

Similarly, problems can arise when a rhesus negative woman becomes pregnant with a rhesus positive foetus. Her body can develop an immune reaction that will prevent her successfully carrying another baby by the same partner. This can be overcome through donor insemination using a rhesus negative donor.

Donor insemination is a relatively simple procedure whereby a frozen semen specimen, which has been selected to match you and your partner's physical characteristics and blood group, is thawed before being inserted into the vagina around the time of ovulation or on successive days to coincide with ovulation. This is usually repeated every month or every other month.

The sperm specimen used is always a thawed, previously frozen one. This is because the specimen must be kept frozen while the donor is assessed for human immunodeficiency virus (HIV). Only when the donor has been found to be free of the virus six months after producing the specimen can the sperm be released from quarantine for use. This is an ongoing process, designed to protect the recipient and any child that may result.

The treatment itself is usually carried out by a doctor or nurse who will place the sperm in the cervical canal. This procedure is painless and takes very little time. The woman may be advised to rest for a short time afterwards and she will be told not to douche or bathe immediately before or after treatment, although some women known to have acidic mucus may be advised to use a bicarbonate of soda douche prior to insemination.

If the clinic doctor is monitoring ovulation, he may suggest that you attend for a further insemination on successive days to ensure that the treatment coincides with ovulation. DI may be combined with ovarian stimulation to increase the number of eggs available for fertilization (see page 84). It is often because of the stress of treatment that couples are advised to have treatment every other month, particularly where ovulation induction is combined with DI, to give them a break between treatments.

The donor

As mentioned earlier, donor semen and blood specimens are screened to eliminate the presence of any infectious diseases and a quarantine is imposed on all specimens while the donor is screened for the HIV virus. Donors, who are often university students, are generally given a small sum of money for each sample, although most donate for altruistic reasons.

There is a move to recruit more donors from among men who have already had a family, as the views of their families regarding the donation can then be taken into account. Although it is inadvisable for you to have a known donor for yourselves, you may like to ask close friends or relatives if they would consider donating sperm to a clinic near their home as it would help couples like yourselves.

Clinics are not allowed to achieve more than ten live births from one donor, which means that they always need more donors, and a shortage of donors may delay treatment still further. If there is a particular cultural, religious, or ethnic background that you require in a donor, this may become even more important. Clinics do not have a limitless supply of donors and may have to contact other clinics to obtain a donor meeting your requirements. In some cases they may not be able to match your requirements at all.

The donor remains anonymous and will never know the outcome of his donation. Similarly, you will never know much more about your donor than his physical characteristics, ethnic background, and genetic history, although donors are being encouraged to give more non-identifying information about themselves for the benefit of any child who may, in time, make enquiries about his or her father. Currently, there is no provision in the law for this. The Human Fertilisation and Embryology Act allows the Government to make regulations covering what information will be made available to children, and the Government has indicated that it will consult widely before doing this. All donors are carefully selected. They are required to be healthy, with no history of hereditary disease, and of reasonable appearance and intelligence.

Once you have been counselled and you feel you fully understand and accept the implications of DI, a suitable donor is selected. Your clinic will primarily try to match your partner's ethnic origin, physical characteristics, and blood group, meeting any special requirements that you may have, such as religious background. It very much depends on the number of donors a clinic has access to as to how much choice they can offer.

Many couples who are successful through DI want to try for a second child with the same donor. This is generally not a problem as the clinic will have a coded record of the donor and should have access to more of that donor's sperm. Also, even if ten live births have already been achieved with that donor, the law allows the number to be exceeded in such a situation.

The clinic is obliged, by law, to send information about donors, recipients, and the outcome of treatment to the HFEA. This is so the use of donated gametes can be monitored and regulated. It ensures that sperm from one donor is not used for more than ten live births, and helps avoid the remote possibility that two children born as a result of clinics using the same donor might wish to marry – though the odds against this happening are enormous!

The potential also exists for any DI child, reaching the age of 18, to providing that the child is aware of their status as a DI child. The current law states that this will not include any identifying information. In the unlikely event that the law changes, your clinic will be legally obliged to inform you about this before commencement of treatment. If the law does ever change, it will not retrospectively affect any children born as a result of treatment given before the law was altered, and it will not affect any donor's anonymity. Any information stored by both the clinic and the Authority is kept secure and completely confidential. Clinics will require you to notify them of the outcome of your treatment so that they can provide the HFEA with the information it is required to keep.

The outcome of DI

In the UK, for the first time, reliable data regarding the number and outcome of DI treatments has been published. In 85 centres during the last 5 months of 1991, 4260 patients underwent 9262 treatment cycles. There was a live birth rate of just under 5 per cent per treatment cycle. This success rate was seen to fall after five attempts from 5.4 to 4.1 per cent and in relation to the age of the woman. Pregnancy rates were relatively similar for women in the 25–39 age group, dropping significantly for women over 39.

Data published in 1994 showed that, in 1992, in 87 centres, 7911 patients underwent over 26 000 treatment cycles with an overall birth rate of 5 per cent per treatment cycle.

Another variable factor in success rate will be the expertise of the clinic. Some clinics may perform more DI than others and so may subsequently achieve greater success, although some smaller clinics may be able to offer more individual care, which may give rise to better results. There is no evidence of any increase in foetal abnormality with a DI pregnancy. It is accepted good practice that the treatment is appraised after five or six attempts without success. Further investigation may be needed before treatment recommences or GIFT or IVF using donor sperm may be the next step.

Approximately 60 per cent of those couples offered DI decide to go ahead with it. To some couples, it is simply unacceptable. Those who do pursue DI feel that, compared with the alternative of adoption, the child would at least be half theirs genetically. Fewer than 1000 babies were placed last year for adoption, so it is probable that there is really no alternative for many couples anyway.

Some women do find the procedure stressful, reporting that they feel that they are being unfaithful to their partner. It is often helpful for you both if you both go to the clinic and share the experience, and some clinics may encourage male partners to assist with the insemination itself.

The most important aspect of this treatment by far is the amount of thought and discussion that takes place before treatment starts. It is vital that you and your partner have full and frank discussions, both together and with a counsellor at the clinic, to help you decide whether or not this is the path you wish to follow. Most couples feel that they cannot commence treatment quickly enough, but doctors are now obliged to give you sufficient time, usually around two months, to consider the implications of treatment before signing the detailed consent form and commencing treatment. If you subsequently change your minds, do not worry, you will be able to postpone or opt out of treatment at any time.

The first consideration is, are you both satisfied that there is no other way that you might have a child of your own – that is, one who is genetically yours and your partner's. Any lingering doubt must be explored before you start. Nothing is ever black and white and there are relatively few cases where a doctor can categorically state that you will never conceive with your partner.

Doctors routinely advise couples considering DI to continue to have intercourse over the duration of treatment. There is a school of thought that this primes the uterus to make it more receptive to sperm. This does, however, cloud the issue. In instances of oligospermia there is always the possibility that the child is the partner's, not the donor's.

Who are you going to tell?

It is important for both you and your partner to fully comprehend the gravity of your action. In the majority of cases, the woman will become pregnant with a child that, genetically, is not her partner's. She will feel sadness that she has not been able to bear his child; he may feel many conflicting emotions. It is really vital, then, for you both to explore these feelings beforehand. Once a pregnancy is established, it is too late for doubts.

Another area that must be considered is that of disclosure. If treatment is successful, you and your partner will share the pregnancy together. No one else need ever know that your partner is not your child's genetic father, and, in every other sense, he will be your child's natural father. After all, being a father is not just a matter of biology. Further, the status of the DI father has been clarified in law. If both partners consented to this treatment, the male partner is recognized in law as being the legal father. This also applies if your partner is *not* married to you, but consents to treatment. The law clearly states that donors have no rights over any children born as a result of their donation. But, would you tell the child that he or she is a result of DI? Would you tell anyone else? The only people who would actually *need* to know are the doctors and clinic staff who treat you and, possibly, your family doctor. If you prefer your family doctor were not told, the clinic is obliged to respect your confidentiality, although there may be medical reasons for your doctor needing to know.

There will be many moments during the life of a child when parental origin is discussed – 'He looks just like his father', 'She is very good at art, who does she take after?', as well as routine medical questions about hereditary diseases. Extended family members will look for likenesses and characteristic traits.

Whether you choose to tell your DI child about his or her origins is entirely up to you. Researchers have found that some DI children are generally aware that 'something is up' – exchanged glances between parents at significant moments, areas where there is a real difference in personality and aptitude, but, in truth, these exist for many children who are not DI children. You must also understand why you have chosen to disclose the fact or not to – is it to protect the child or is it to protect yourselves?

Secrets can be harmful and dangerous. Parents can be on a knife-edge about the secret getting out. Children who do find out accidentally or late in life may feel that they have been misled or lied to. One woman, who was ultimately told by her mother after the death of her social father, felt cheated that she had never been given the opportunity to tell him that she loved him and that she regarded him as her real father in every sense.

Letting *some* people in on a secret does not mean telling *everyone*. You may begin to tell the child as they grow to an age where they can begin to understand – perhaps five or six – answering questions as they arise over the ensuing years. Most children can accept these disclosures well because, as far as they are concerned, this is not out of the ordinary. As the child grows older, they will understand just how much they were wanted, that you were prepared to go to such great lengths to have them.

There are quite a considerable number of children now who are, openly or otherwise, not the genetic offspring of the husband or partner of their mother. There is no shame in having a DI child. Perhaps the most difficult issue to explain to a child is the anonymity of the donor, that they will never know who their genetic father was. For this reason, donors are encouraged to give more information, such as interests, talents, some family background, and anything else of a non-identifying nature that might prove helpful to children seeking more information in the future. These issues are explored in *The Gift of a Child*, by Snowden and Snowden.

You may also feel that it would be helpful to talk to another couple who have a DI child. ISSUE and CHILD should be able to put you in touch with other couples in your area who will be happy to share their experiences, although most good clinics have their own patient support group (see page 144 for addresses).

Ovum donation

It is now possible for eggs to be donated to infertile couples, just as sperm is donated. This is helpful for those women who are unable to produce eggs themselves, through ovulatory failure, or removal of the ovaries, chemotherapy, or conditions such as Turner's Syndrome, where the ovaries never develop fully.

There are also women who are carriers of inherited disorders, such as Duchennes muscular dystrophy. If these women give birth to a child who inherits the disorder, it may suffer greatly and die at an early age. This risk is removed if the woman achieves pregnancy with a donated egg. Egg donation may also be of benefit to older women, giving them a better chance of pregnancy.

Unfortunately, eggs are a lot less easy than sperm to collect and there are always fewer donors available than there are potential recipients, so waiting lists for donor eggs are very long. It is also unfortunate that, at the time of writing, no method exists of freezing unfertilized eggs satisfactorily.

One way doctors have obtained eggs for donation is from women who already have a family and who seek operative sterilization to prevent them having any more children. These women and their partners are counselled by the doctor and asked whether they would be prepared to undergo ovarian stimulation prior to their operation so that egg collection can be performed simultaneously.

Many couples are willing to help childless couples in this way without any reward. Some women are thus able to have their operation performed privately at no cost to themselves.

There is a small group of women who already have a family, who have elected to go through the process of ovarian stimulation and egg collection simply so that they can donate their eggs to couples less fortunate than themselves.

It would be inappropriate for such women to be paid large sums of money for this service as no woman should undergo an operation needlessly or for money. There are risks attached to both ovarian stimulation and egg collection, so it is understandable that there are not many donors.

Occasionally, couples undergoing IVF or GIFT may donate any spare eggs to other couples, but the fact that these eggs can be inseminated and frozen for them to try again usually means that few are available.

One issue currently being debated is whether or not a relative or friend should be allowed to donate eggs. This usually applies to sisters, but it has been known in mothers and daughters, too! The arguments for and against this are considerable.

Feelings are mixed about the wisdom of using a known ovum donor. Many women feel that a baby derived from their sister's egg at least shares their own genetic makeup. This is an enormous gift for one woman to give another, but the subsequent relationship between the two women may suffer some strain, as both may feel that they have some parental rights over the child and its upbringing, and this may cause confusion for the resulting child, too.

Known donation is permissible in law, but, in practice, many clinics prefer that potential recipients recruit donors who will donate for other, unknown couples, thereby increasing the number of donors available and shortening the waiting list for all.

Controversially, a small number of clinics in the UK will offer free fertility treatment to those patients who are prepared to donate some of their eggs to other couples. This is obviously a very sensitive issue, requiring thorough counselling, and, in fact, relatively few couples feel that, in the absence of a child of their own, they are prepared to make such a donation.

As a result of the fact that there are still far more women requiring ovum donation than there are eggs available, doctors have been looking at alternative sources of human ova. Two possible sources have been identified, eggs obtained from aborted foetal material and eggs obtained from a cadaver, in the same way that vital organs are currently donated following the death of the donor.

Following extensive public consultation, the HFEA concluded in 1994 that the use of foetal ovarian tissue in fertility treatment was not acceptable. Also, although the Authority did not object in principle to the use of cadaveric ovarian tissue from adult women, it decided not to approve its use.

Children born as a result of sperm or ovum donation today will know (if their parents choose to inform them of their origins in the future) that their genetic parents made a conscious, considered, and informed decision to donate their genetic material to create a new life. Basic non-identifying information about all such donors can be made available by the HFEA should the child wish to seek it.

Egg donors are treated in law the same way as are sperm donors. The name of the donor is never passed on to the recipients or their children, although the clinic has to notify the HFEA of the names of the donor, the recipients, and the outcome of treatment. Similarly, the HFEA allows a limit of ten live births to be achieved using any one donor.

Ovum donors are screened for diseases such as hepatitis B and HIV and questioned about hereditary diseases and medical history. If a donor deliberately withholds information about hereditary disease and a child is subsequently born as a result of ovum donation with a disability that a donor should reasonably have known about, the donor may be legally liable.

The woman receiving treatment and her partner or husband are regarded in law as the legal parents of any child that may be born as a result of treatment. The donor has no rights over the child and the child has no claim on the donor.

Ovum donation – where the sperm used is the partner's sperm – seems to be less problematical psychologically for the couple than sperm donation, in that the woman receives a fertilized egg, becomes pregnant, delivers the baby, and bonds with it in the same way as any other mother.

♀ ♂ Surrogacy

Surrogacy refers to an arrangement whereby another woman, usually unrelated to both partners, makes a contract to bear a child and give it to the childless couple. This is only appropriate where a woman has no uterus or is unable to sustain a pregnancy. The HFEA Code of Practice does not permit doctors to assist a surrogacy arrangement for reasons of convenience, say, where a woman would like a child but does not wish to go through a pregnancy! Surrogacy arrangements are permitted where it is physically impossible or medically undesirable for the commissioning mother to carry a baby to full term.

There are some women who enjoy pregnancy, although they perhaps do not wish for another child. It is such a woman who might consider becoming a surrogate mother.

It is illegal to offer the surrogacy arrangement for any commercial gain, although it is permissible for reasonable expenses to be paid.

There are a number of possible permutations of surrogacy, with the surrogate mother having no genetic relationship to the foetus, which might be the result of either donated sperm and egg, or sperm and egg from both commissioning partners. It is also possible for the surrogate mother to be inseminated artificially by the commissioning father, so that she is the genetic mother.

Surrogacy is legally permitted, providing no commercial arrangement is entered into by the participants. The most common form of surrogacy is organized through a specialist, licensed clinic by IVF, where eggs are collected from the commissioning mother, fertilized by her partner and replaced in the surrogate mother.

A great deal of counselling is required before such an undertaking can be entered into by both the commissioning couple and the surrogate mother and her family. The most difficult part of such treatment is when the surrogate mother comes to hand over the baby she has carried for nine months. There have been widely publicized cases where the surrogate mother has felt unable to give up the child, even though she entered into the arrangement knowing that this would be the end result. This is less likely when the sperm and egg used come from the commissioning couple.

Providing all parties are agreed, an application has to be made to the courts, within six months of the birth, before the commissioning parents can become the legal parents of the child. This is currently under review, as the Government is issuing regulations making power for 'Parental Orders' in surrogacy arrangements involving licensed treatments, known as 'fast track' adoption arrangements. This is intended to speed up and clarify the process.

If you feel that you would like to know more about surrogacy, contact Kim Cotton or Gena Dodds at COTS (Childlessness Overcome through Surrogacy) – their address is given on page 144.

♀ ♂ *Pre-implantation diagnosis*

The considerable progress that has been made in embryo research since the passage of the Human Fertilisation and Embryology Act has made it possible to examine a human embryo when it is only a few days old by removing a single cell or two without subsequent damage to the embryo.

Using just one or two cells, scientists can determine the sex of the embryo. As some serious inherited diseases are only passed on through children of one sex, embryos of that sex can be discarded, and only those that can be predicted to be of the unaffected sex are replaced.

In time, it is hoped that continued research will enable doctors to identify all those embryos that might be affected by a serious, life-threatening hereditary condition before implantation, to allow couples who are carriers to have unaffected children. This research brings great hope to families affected by haemophilia, sickle cell anaemia, and cystic fibrosis.

There is some public concern that pre-implantation diagnosis may be developed for more trivial reasons, such as sex selection for purely social purposes or the pursuit of the perfect child. However, it is unlikely that any couple would subject themselves to the trauma, stress, and expense of IVF unless they had to, and even more unlikely that any right-minded doctor would support them in such a quest.

6

How to choose a clinic

♀ ♂ *The options*

Most district general hospitals can offer basic infertility investigation and treatment up to ovulation induction and artificial insemination using a partner's sperm. Some may offer tubal surgery and tubal microsurgery, while others may provide treatment, including egg collection and GIFT.

It is now necessary for any clinic providing more intensive services, including DI and IVF or any treatment involving the collection and storage of eggs or sperm or the creation of embryos, to hold a licence granted by the HFEA. There are currently just over 100 such clinics throughout the UK.

The majority of subfertile couples can be helped to conceive at the district hospital if they do not manage, in time, to do so on their own. If, however, time is passing by without a satisfactory conclusion being reached, many couples start to feel that they should be looking elsewhere for help.

How soon this happens depends on the age of the couple, particularly the woman, how long you have been trying, and how helpful your district hospital has been.

If you are over 30, have been trying for more than a couple of years, and feel that you have exhausted all the local facilities, you may feel that it is time to seek referral to a specialist centre. Even though you may not require advanced treatments, such as IVF or DI, it is likely that a specialist centre will have the facilities required to diagnose the reason for your subfertility accurately and treat it appropriately. In addition, licensed centres are obliged to make counselling available to all couples. This is particularly valuable in helping you come to terms with your subfertility and cope with the pressures of treatment.

If you have spent some time trying to have a baby without success, you may, however, feel that enough is enough – you will accept your subfertility, come to terms with it, and get on with your life. In time, you might become pregnant, but, if not, you will know you tried your best. You may like to look at other options, such as adoption, or you may start to face up to the idea of life without children. Good counselling is invaluable at this time.

113

Some men and women feel driven, however, to leave no stone unturned in their quest for a family. Before reading the rest of this chapter, please take some time to consider this point. If you persist with further treatment or investigation, you will undoubtedly put yourselves through a lot of stress, pain, and, perhaps, disappointment. You may incur considerable expense, your relationship with your partner and your career may come under intense strain, and you may not end up with the baby you so desire.

Even if you do become pregnant, there may be considerations you have not taken into account. Multiple pregnancies, of twins, triplets, or more, are a common result of assisted conception treatment. Over a quarter of IVF pregnancies result in twins.

How far are you prepared to go? Ideally you want your own baby by your own partner, but at what point would you consider using a donor for sperm, for an egg, or both? How much of your life are you prepared to spend having blood tests, injections, or surgery in your quest to become parents?

Some couples have described the ongoing process of investigation and treatment against the rapid ticking of the biological clock as a treadmill, which it becomes increasingly difficult to step off. Although the information that follows is designed to help you find the best treatment for you, only you can decide how far you will go.

If you or your clinic doctor feel that you have nothing more to gain from attending your local clinic – perhaps you feel that delays between appointments have led to precious time slipping away or there is nothing more they can do for you – you will require referral to a specialist clinic.

Surprisingly, there is little NHS funding for specialist subfertility care and, indeed, some patients may find they even have to meet the costs of some basic investigations, drugs, and treatment at their local hospital. Even though many of the licensed clinics are situated within NHS hospitals, only two (at the time of writing) have full funding from the NHS; the remainder require that patients meet some or all of the costs of investigation and treatment. In addition to the NHS based clinics, there are a large number of wholly private, licensed clinics.

It may be preferable to seek further treatment through the NHS first as it is likely to be less expensive than private centres, and it will help ensure that NHS administrators are aware of the demand for these services. For some couples, however, perhaps because of age or the existence of other children in the family, appropriate NHS treatment is simply not available.

Changes within the NHS may also make it more difficult to gain access to such treatment as District Health Authorities are forced to prioritize health care. Subfertility is rarely regarded as a high priority, even though it accounts for a large proportion of patients under 40 who are referred to hospital.

There are far more private clinics offering advanced subfertility management than there are NHS programmes. This has arisen largely because the NHS cannot meet the cost of developing the technology required, and also because the waiting lists at many NHS clinics have grown so long that many women feel they just cannot wait that long.

To go to one of the private clinics, you will require a letter of referral from either your GP or clinic doctor. The more information that can be supplied, the less investigation will be required at the new clinic. Some clinics will liaise with your local doctor if you live far away and arrange for some of your tests to be conducted nearer to home.

Your referring doctor may recommend a clinic with which they have had previous contact, although this may be because they know little about any others, or they may give you a selection to choose from. You should still conduct your own survey as your doctor is unlikely to mind if you ask to be referred to another clinic of your choice.

Although the information given here refers principally to private clinics as some of the NHS clinics charge fees on a par with private clinics, it can be taken to apply to both. The choice of NHS clinics may be limited as they may only accept patients from a given catchment area. Those that receive some NHS funding generally have very long waiting lists (sometimes it is over two years before the next available appointment).

If you are lucky enough to be accepted on to the waiting list of such a clinic and don't want to wait so long for treatment, many of them accept fee-paying patients in the shorter term as a means of subsidizing the treatment of the others. You may be able to afford one or two private attempts at treatment while you are on the waiting list. If you are successful, the waiting list is shortened; if not, at least the clinic has secured some funding towards your own eventual treatment.

It is not generally a good idea to seek private treatment elsewhere while on an NHS waiting list without discussing it with the clinic beforehand. If, however, the NHS clinic has no private facility and the waiting list is considerable, it is understandable that you might want to seek more prompt attention, if you can afford it, in the meantime.

Shopping around between clinics may prove costly and confusing as some clinics may insist on repeating assessments already completed elsewhere. In addition, each clinic has its own methods, which may unsettle you if they seem contrary to what you expect. None the less, by shopping around you may also find a clinic that suits your needs better.

♀ ♂ *How much will private treatment cost?*

If you have private health insurance, check beforehand whether you are covered for 'fertility' investigations. Very few insurers offer to meet the costs of IVF or GIFT and some may not even cover investigations for subfertility or for a condition in existence before the policy was taken out.

Can you afford private treatment? It is very expensive and there is no guarantee that you will be successful. It is inadvisable to borrow money or spend more than you can afford; some couples have spent more than £10 000 with no baby at the end.

Although all clinics have their own price list, you can expect IVF or GIFT to cost over a thousand pounds per attempt. Some, which operate from NHS premises, are able to charge considerably less. Basic investigations, such as blood tests and semen analyses, as well as medical consultations, are not usually included in the price of a treatment cycle.

It may not be possible to find a clinic within easy reach of your home. Consider the cost of travelling to the clinic and also the cost of accommodation in the area, as it is likely that you and your partner may have to stay away for at least one night. It might be more appropriate to find a clinic near to where friends or family live, as you then might be able to stay with them.

What will you have to pay for?

Ask for a full list of prices, to include:

- first and subsequent medical consultations
- standard pre-IVF and GIFT investigations
- diagnostic laparoscopy
- full IVF or GIFT cycle.

The costs for a full cycle should cover all ultrasound scans, blood and urine tests, egg collection, and, for IVF, embryo transfer. It is not usual to find that the cost of ovarian stimulation drugs have been included. If, for any reason, a treatment cycle is postponed before reaching egg collection or embryo transfer, the clinic should re-imburse you some part of your original fee – how much should be agreed beforehand.

Ask if the price of a full cycle includes the cost of a consultation with one of the doctors in the event of failure, to discuss future options. Ask also if counselling costs are included in the fee quoted.

If you have been referred for GIFT or IVF, the clinic doctor may insist on performing a diagnostic laparoscopy before proceeding with treatment. This adds to the cost and time of treatment, but it may be very important. In some cases, your referring doctor may be able to do this for you locally. Check the clinic's policy on this beforehand.

Good clinics will require evidence that thorough investigations have been carried out to identify the cause of your subfertility. These should include an X-ray of the womb (hysterosalpingogram) and thorough semen analysis. If these have not been done recently, do not be surprised if clinics insist that they be performed or repeated; this will increase the full cost of treatment.

Ask for a full list of available facilities.

Unless your referring doctor is convinced that you need IVF or GIFT you may require other, less invasive treatments, but some clinics cannot provide these. If there is a possibility you may require DI, check that the clinic is licensed to offer this.

If IVF is likely to be appropriate, ask how they do it. It is not always necessary to have a general anaesthetic. Can the clinic offer what you want? Clinics collecting eggs under sedation only may be less expensive. Is the treatment cycle monitored thoroughly, with blood or urine tests to measure the hormones that vitally affect the outcome?

There have been reports of couples undergoing IVF where eggs fail to fertilize due to temporarily poor-quality sperm. There is no excuse for clinics offering treatment without first performing a routine semen analysis. This simple procedure could prevent a woman being put through the severe physical and emotional trauma of treatment when there is little hope of success at that time. Treatment should be delayed until sperm quality is confirmed. Check that the clinic does this *every time*.

Eggs that are difficult to retrieve through the laparoscope can be collected with the use of ultrasound. Check that the clinic is able to perform *both* methods of collection.

♀ ♂ *Which is the best clinic for you?*

Before deciding on a clinic, be sure that you know what you require. Relatively few patients need assisted conception treatment. If less invasive treatments might be appropriate for you, do not choose a clinic that only offers IVF – find a clinic that provides full investigations and a full range of treatments.

Those looking for GIFT treatment may prefer to seek treatment at a clinic that is a licensed IVF centre that also offers GIFT, rather than one not providing IVF. Not only will the clinic have passed the scrutiny of the licensing authority, but it is more likely to have the capacity to freeze any spare embryos produced.

Identify five or so clinics that you feel you can get to fairly easily and make a list of questions you are going to ask each one before telephoning them. Not only are the answers to your questions important, but also the way in which your enquiry is handled. Is there a helpful person there who is prepared to talk to you when you call or, if they are busy, are they prepared to call you back? Are they reluctant for you to visit the centre to look around? You can compare the results of your calls before reducing your list to around three clinics, which you should take time to visit.

You will be placing an enormous investment – both financial and emotional – in the clinic you settle on, so it makes sense that you should have a good look at each one before deciding. Are the staff friendly? Did you feel confident with the team? Did they have time to spend with you, showing you around, or were they too busy? Does this mean that they will be too busy to answer your questions when you are their patient?

If they have too much time and the clinic seems very quiet, perhaps there aren't many other patients. This may mean they have plenty of time for each patient, but it may also indicate that this is a very small clinic and the smaller clinics have consistently returned poorer results than the larger, more busy clinics.

What facilities are there for patients? Is there a patient support group? Why not talk to some of the others in the waiting room to see if they are happy with the service they are receiving.

You should also look at any literature the clinic provides. Is it clear and comprehensive or just glossy and expensive with little information? Are adequate facilities available for independent counselling – a vital part of subfertility management? You may also want to see what facilities are available for men to produce semen samples. This is very important for men who do not feel happy having to perform in a loo in a busy corridor.

Some clinics offering a private service within an NHS hospital do not have a lavish environment to offer patients. In fact, very often, the facilities are no different from those on offer to NHS patients, the only difference being that there is not the delay of the waiting list. These clinics are likely to be slightly less expensive than strictly private clinics and some patients prefer to attend such a clinic, knowing that profits go directly back into the NHS. Incidentally, a lot of the research required to maintain the improvements in treatment is conducted in these underfunded units.

Success rates

By far the most important question most couples want answered is how successful the clinic is in helping women become pregnant. Some clinics are much more successful than others in achieving pregnancies and *independent* information to help you establish which clinics these are is vital. Obviously every private clinic wants your business and this may prompt them to give you the most promising picture of their success rates. If the clinic quotes a success rate of 30 per cent, is this perhaps 30 per cent of *all* patients or 30 per cent of a *selected group*, whose chances of success may be greater?

Furthermore, clinics may be happy to report success rates in terms of *pregnancies*, some of which may not reach term, or in terms of numbers of *babies* born, which may include those born as twins or triplets, so it is important to be clear what their success rate refers to.

The HFEA plans to make available to patients information concerning results achieved in individual centres which enables patients to judge which clinic will best suit their needs.

One means by which you can assess success rates is to ask each clinic what success they have achieved over the last 12 months with women of a similar age and diagnosis group as yourselves. Ask also for the total number of women treated and the results based on the number of embryos or eggs returned or DI cycles. This will help you decide which is the most successful. If a clinic is reluctant to give you this information, you will have to consider why this might be.

The results achieved by a clinic may vary considerably as some may not treat women over a given age, say 38 or 40 years old. These clinics are more likely to have a better overall success rate than a clinic that treats older women. It is, however, the individual success rate in relation to your own circumstances that is most important.

In general, the overall success rate for IVF is between 10 and 20 per cent per embryo transfer. For GIFT, overall success rates are around 20–25 per cent per patient.

Results for all centres and all IVF patients, irrespective of age and causative factor as reported to the HFEA, for 1992 show a live birth rate of 12.7 per cent per treatment cycle. This is somewhat lower than the rate in 1991, of 13.9 per cent, which may be attributable to an increase in the average age of women undergoing IVF to 34.

Other questions to ask

Ask what provision the clinic makes for bank holidays and weekends. This is to avoid the considerable disappointment that might follow if you have been prepared for egg collection only to find that there is no doctor available on the day to do it.

You should also ask how long you will have to wait for treatment. If you choose a clinic because you wish to be seen by a particular doctor you may have to wait longer. Don't expect treatment – even private treatment – to commence straight away as there is often some delay while information is gathered from referring doctors or just because the clinic has a waiting list.

If you are unhappy with the treatment you receive at any clinic, your GP can refer you to another clinic without too much difficulty. You should also notify the HFEA if you feel that your treatment was unsatisfactory.

The HFEA is primarily funded from license fees charged to clinics for treatment cycles, £40 per IVF cycle and £10 per DI cycle, charges that are generally passed directly on to the patients.

You can obtain a complete list of licensed clinics from the HFEA, along with several very helpful information leaflets (for their address see page 144). In addition, clinics have available a video produced by the HFEA on both IVF and DI that they can lend to you to view at home.

7

The emotional cost

To so many outsiders it may seem as if the subfertile simply go through two stages: trying for a baby, then discovering it's impossible. You live in hope, then your hope is either realized or dashed.

But, of course, as you know, it isn't like this. There is a high emotional price to pay for being subfertile. Because of the extraordinary advances in treatments, hopes are very rarely dashed, except in cases where a woman has had a total hysterectomy and the man's sperm count is nil. And even then, there is usually always another last-ditch option waiting round the corner, even when all other chances have died. To live in hope is to live in a kind of hell, as many of you will have already found out.

First, there is the sheer humiliation of all the tests and treatments. Other people have invaded your private space. Their hands have not only reached parts of your body that other hands have never reached, but doctors and nurses in white coats, complete strangers, have stared up you, down you, goggled at your specimens, and asked about the regularity and quality of one of the most intimate aspects of your lives together – your sex life. Couples often feel emotionally abused, even though they have submitted themselves willingly to the abuse in order to reach their goals.

Then there is the sheer physical exhaustion of the tests. Couples may have had to get up at the crack of dawn for days running, travel hundreds of miles, and wait for hours in clinic waiting rooms, often in extreme discomfort or embarrassment. At the end of various treatments, they may be given bad news. Sometimes the tests and treatment can feel like psychological torture, however much, at another level, they are welcomed. The knowledge, too, that while you are undergoing these tests, other people are having children easily, and not appreciating them makes the whole procedure even more painful, as the poignant poem, 'Tests', by Franziska, and the letter that follows show:

I had a dream . . .
I've just given birth
to the most wonderful creation on earth
A girl or boy

Who cares? We've so much joy!

Then I awake
It's all a mistake . . .
There's never been a baby at all
Our only baby is many injections of Pergonal,
(They're so happy – first postnatal clinic is beginning
Her delight, her second toddler is swimming.)

Conceive a child?
I might as well have had a hysterectomy!
(His fourth child is a burden . . . too quick after his
   vasectomy.)
Our momentary three miracles of life, three embryos didn't
   implant.
(Their three miracles of life, cruelly beaten,
now all fostered by an aunt.)

Our teenager is painful catheters, speculums;
eggs and sperm under microscopes
(Their teenager is real and living;
not endless disappointment and dashed hopes . . .)

I had a nightmare
Our child will never get here,
despite spending a fortune on its
transport fare.

I never wanted children and was so glad that we never 'had to' get
married, that we could wait a year or two to start a family,
expecting that it would only take a year at the latest – how wrong I
was! And now five years on the endless trips to the hospital, the
blood tests – I've had so many my veins are clogging. They've even
taken it out of my ankle. The hundreds of tablets I've taken and
what seems like thousands of injections I'd had, that I feel like a
pincushion. How can I feel complete hate for another human just
because she's pregnant (even if we've only just met?) Why do my
family and friends have pleasure in telling me someone I know is
pregnant? They used to tell me 'You're still young, you've got
plenty of time'. They've stopped telling me now because the time
is running out.

    When I started trying I always imagined I'd have a little girl with
long, dark hair, I would call her Laura, she'd be so beautiful I'd be

able to dress her in pretty dresses and plait her hair, but life isn't like that. Instead of the happy noisy house I want, it's quiet. I just want to die and get away from this cruel hard world. How much longer can we carry on? Is it going to be this way for ever till I die?

Not everyone feels quite so bad, of course. There can be great relief in the clinic, knowing that you're not alone. Everyone sitting there is almost certainly in the same boat as you are:

The treatment really isn't that awful. Probably the worst part is the waiting in between each procedure. It pays to keep yourselves occupied during this time and carry on as normally as possible (easier said than done, I know!) I was lucky enough to have a very understanding employer.

A lot of time will be spent in waiting rooms for treatment in hospital, and blood tests and injections at the doctor's. Arm yourself with a good book, newspaper or favourite magazines to pass the time (magazines in waiting rooms are always months out of date!) It's a good idea to take a drink with you and, if you're travelling a long way to hospital, some food to keep your strength up! You will probably see the same people waiting with you each time you go to hospital and there's nothing like a smile and a cheery 'hello' to break the ice . . .

Unless you are one of the very lucky ones, who have treatment and then become pregnant quickly, most subfertile couples will know all about the 'little deaths', for subfertility often involves a dreadful series of small losses. First, there is the feeling of loss every month, when a period comes. But then often bigger hopes are dashed. Perhaps you might become, technically, pregnant, but the pregnancy only lasts a few days. Even if you are lucky enough to become pregnant, it doesn't mean that you will necessarily bring that baby to term. The following women's agonizing cases show how bitterly unhappy, lonely, and, indeed, guilty, they can feel:

At lunchtime today my period started. I cannot explain the feelings of disappointment, sadness, etc. that I feel. I am devastated. If only my period had come earlier I am sure it would have been easier, maybe not. I honestly didn't think it would fail – *why?* I was so convinced this IVF attempt would work, I just am not prepared for this. I couldn't feel worse if I had been pregnant

123

and miscarried. How am I going to tell everyone, how I wish we hadn't told anyone. I have let my husband down, my parents, and all the staff on the unit, once again I am a failure. What have I done wrong in life to deserve this?

Later I received a phone call from the unit asking if I had started as they hadn't heard from me, told them I had, the consultant asked me how I felt and I said: 'Fine'. Why did I say that? I am not fine, I feel dreadful.

Today has to be one of the worst. Yet again I know my treatment has failed. I'm getting period pains. How I hate writing those words. I just hate my body. I hate my life. I hate everything. I hate these feelings of being cheated by life and nature. How I wish I could have died at birth so not have all this pain now. I just can't go through another set of injections. How I long to hold a tiny baby of my own, watch it grow up to see it go to school, to hear it call me mummy, but I know I will never know that phrase that so many people take for granted. If I could I would ask if there is a God to take me now to live in Heaven to get away from this pain. I want to ask my body why? What's so wrong that you can't even get pregnant just once, that's all I ask?

The young 'uns died today – day 6, our fifth IVF attempt – the first frozen/thaw embryo replacement after four fresh attempts. I felt them die and said a silent goodbye whilst walking arm in arm with Mike around our village. It was nine in the evening on a beautiful night.

Just a small twinge, a slight pull in the left lower abdomen and they were gone.

And then there is the even greater loss – the miscarriage. True, those who have had miscarriages at least have the power to become pregnant, you may think, but imagine having a miscarriage at the fourth IVF attempt. Perhaps you have told everyone, and your entire family is celebrating, knitting, and looking forward to you giving birth. At least those previous little deaths were private. A miscarriage, usually, is more public. And yet, still other people, because they have not experienced your joy, or the feeling of carrying your baby inside, cannot identify with you and find it hard to help.

As with the death of a close relative, it is the following months of grieving that are the hardest to deal with. I felt numbed and relieved all at the same time that it was all over but as time passed by, feelings of anger, resentment and a sense of failure all overwhelmed me. I have felt absolute hatred at times of pregnant women all bloomy and happily expectant, and I have been unable to look at a baby in a pram. I have called it the 'empty arms' syndrome. Then has come the guilt, especially when some well-meaning person has pointed out the fact that I already have two lovely girls and that I should count my blessings. Frankly I have found it hard to take. The lack of support after a miscarriage is unbelievable.

I feel as if I'm being punished for at first not wanting my first baby. There isn't a day when I don't feel depressed and cry.

I'm so depressed I can't even sleep. I missed my baby so much I wanted to be with my baby so I took an overdose of Paracematol, but a friend found me and took me to hospital where I saw a psychiatrist who was very nice. But I still can't cope with my feelings. I just bottle them up. I can't snap out of this depression and it seems to get worse every day. I feel everyone is against me because of my mood swings. I blame myself so much thinking that I might have been able to have prevented it, like, what if I didn't go out that day, would I have still carried it? I ask myself every question, over and over again, torturing myself. It has been five months since the miscarriage but only seems five days. Everyone tells me I am still young but it doesn't matter. I am trying to find the strength to carry on, but it is difficult, especially when you've lost a baby that you thought was yours to keep and not let anyone take it away from you as it was a part of you. A part of me is lost with my baby, a part of me that I may never find. My heart is broken and I'm trying to find the missing piece. Every time I hear the song 'Tears in Heaven' by Eric Clapton it reminds me of my baby and my grief.

Eric Clapton, who lost his son when he fell from a New York window, did a great service by talking so publicly as a bereaved father. He brought attention to the grief that men feel when children die. Men are so often left out. And in no area is this highlighted so vividly as in the area of subfertility. Because women bear the brunt of so much testing and treatment, the men's role tends to be forgotten, their feelings ignored, and they can start to feel like mere sperm machines.

But even though they experience fewer tests and treatment, men often find these far more difficult than women. Because of their sex, because of monthly periods, smear tests, even the odd infection like thrush or cystitis, women are much more used to having their sexual parts examined than men. They may suppress their angry feelings because they feel helpless in that stirrupped chair, but at least they are likely to be familiar with it all. Men, though, can find examination or being asked for sperm samples incredibly humiliating. Some men simply refuse, and the fertility tests end there. They would literally rather not have a baby than have a test.

Men often feel threatened, embarrassed, and left out of the fertility merry-go-round, and are far more likely to get angry – with doctors, clinics, nurses, or the system generally.

If it turns out that the man is the infertile one in the partnership, often the woman, according to Jennifer Hunt, takes responsibility for making things easier for him: 'You get more sympathy if you're a woman,' she says, 'but when I counsel couples, men seem to be just as upset as the women. Luckily, the couple often take it in turns to feel unhappy while the other is being strong.'

Obviously, if the man is the infertile one, the woman is left with her fertility and may feel like having an affair, just to become pregnant. Men's reactions vary, perhaps becoming impotent or, alternatively, highly sexual. 'But if we are talking to a man about his infertility, we would never mention AID in the same breath', says Jennifer Hunt. 'That would be like saying you're infertile, but hey presto here's Arnold Schwarzenegger with his amazing sperm. We simply say: "Do you want to discuss alternatives?" They know what we mean.' Mr Z, who wrote the following, felt that he was treated like an 'invisible man' when it came to tests and treatment, and his letter reflects his fury at the powerlessness and degradation he feels about everything, from doctors to booklets. Though no doubt his feelings are justified, the intensity of the anger coming from the letter surely stems, to some extent, from the fact that he and his partner are subfertile:

Thanks to the doctors and clinics I have had to deal with since I discovered we had a fertility problem I know who I am: the Invisible Man. I am administratively an appendage of my wife – who in any case is the one who must undergo nearly all the examinations, invasions and pain in our efforts to have a child. Since we have different surnames, my files are kept under her name and not mine: for the clinics I'm not sure that I exist at all, except to 'consent'. They are certainly put out by my presence, though so far I have always been 'allowed in' with my wife when we've been for a consultation (though once this meant the doctor having to stand as there were only two chairs in the room!)

Insensitivity isn't the word for it. Where is that sense, which those nice books for couples with fertility problems insist on, that infertility is a joint problem and both partners have to be treated together? For the doctors, I don't appear to have feelings at all. One very senior consultant asked my wife, in front of me: 'Have you been exposed to any other males?' Does he do that with every couple? Does he think the woman will never lie to protect herself or her partner's feelings when he is there beside her? In many years of working with couples, could he not have found a way of asking this question which acknowledged the presence – and feelings – of the man? Or does he leave the 'soppy stuff' to the clinic counsellor?

Nor does it get better when you come to things in print. A leaflet on artificial insemination – recently revised – supposedly addresses the couple. But read on! 'A doctor or nurse will insert a simple instrument into your vagina.' Do I have a vagina? I do not, and this could come as a surprise to a doctor or nurse. But that's not the point. It's just that I have become invisible again. But who cares? After all, most infertility experts are gynaecologists. Their careers are built on treating women, not men. Why should they bother about some man with a fragile ego, and even more fragile sperm?

My wife and I have always had an understanding that this was our problem and she has never reproached me, not once, even though she has borne nearly all the physical pain and discomfort of probes, anaesthetics, injections and long-distance travel. Why can the doctors and clinics not see it as a shared problem too? I don't accompany my wife to the clinic for a 'treat'. I am not a little boy who has to sit quietly while his mummy talks to the doctor. I am not, in spite of what they would like to be the case, an Invisible Man.

Subfertility puts an enormous strain on partnerships. And seeing whether it can take such stress is a good test of the strength of the partnership. Some couples do break up; some couples become closer; some stay much the same. But, though it is a joint problem and one that is best borne together, this is advice easier given than taken. Sometimes couples feel like two playing cards, leaning on each other. If one gives way, the other collapses too. If one can be strong while the other is weak and take it in turns, fine, but what if both break down together? The loneliness that each partner can feel is acute. Even grandparents sometimes find it hard to be strong because they, too, feel loss and may not wish to speak of the matter because it upsets them so much.

You will also find couples in which one person bears the grief and anger for the other – usually the woman. If the man were able to admit to his own feelings of loss and anguish just now and again, how much better the woman would feel! But, because the feelings are too painful for him, and because he has been taught not to cry, the woman finds herself bearing all the pain and bitterness for both of them, often becoming labelled almost neurotic in her despair.

Certainly, there will be few couples who don't find subfertility a strain on their sex lives. Sometimes a man simply won't be able to perform at the right time of the month. Alternatively, although he may be intellectually willing, his emotions – angry with being what he feels 'ordered about' by a clinic's advice or a partner desperate to become pregnant – simply refuse to cooperate, making sex impossible. Men who complain that they feel simply like a stud when it comes to sex in this situation, should be reminded that it's no fun for women either, who may also find sex at prescribed times, whether they feel sexy or not, a humiliating chore that makes them feel like a mere incubator. Performing at certain times of the month may also have a bad effect on a couple's sex life in the future; it becomes so much of a timed event that couples may well be making quite clinical appointments for sex, even after their fertility problems have been resolved one way or another. The following couples found the going hard:

We started to argue. It put a big strain on our marriage. You argue about anything because you are under such emotional stress and strain. You blame each other. John began saying: 'If you were a girl from the East End and didn't think about it all the time, you'd get pregnant.'

I knew I couldn't really blame him. Soon after we started investigations, it became clear that the problem lay with me, not him. But he didn't understand how I felt. He said he wanted children, but he didn't take it as far as me.

After three years of trying I became obsessed by it. In the end I couldn't think about anything else. Getting pregnant was my top priority in life because everybody else could do it so easily. I had to do it if it killed me. I was so demoralized. In the end I just wanted to die more than anything else in the world. I wanted to commit suicide but coward that I am I couldn't do it myself.

I told my husband to leave me. I thought he could have a child if he was with someone else but he told me I was stupid and that he had married me because he loved me, not for the children we might have. He wouldn't talk about it.

My husband and I are going through a bad patch at the moment, having recently experienced a failed IVF attempt. It has left me in a state of acute anxiety and although I have had all the support in the world from my husband, I am having great difficulty in bouncing back, so many times in the past I have been rock-bottom but this time I'm the first to admit I feel absolutely desperate. Apart from the feeling of total isolation, which I know is common among infertile couples, I've also lost all my self-confidence which has caused me to appear very unfriendly towards people who even have the remotest connection with children. I suppose it's a mixture of jealousy and envy; either way it's so unlike me and I'm frightened my whole personality is changing. Everyone says they understand but I don't see how they can unless they've experienced the pain and the emotional anguish. Little did I know when this nightmare started seven years ago how it was going to affect me.

Everything in the garden seemed to be perfect then, when after three years of marriage we felt the time was right to start a family. I'd always adored children and my husband felt the same so we felt it wouldn't be too long before that much-wanted little bundle was placed in our proud arms. About this time, our brothers and sisters-in-law, unbeknown to us, were also trying for a baby. They both fell very quickly and had beautiful little boys. Our months of trying were already turning into one whole year of disappointments . . . People keep telling us that it's not the end of the world – you still have each other. I hasten to add that all of these people have had a choice of whether to have a child of their own – that's the difference.

When we found my partner had a problem, the specialist said 'What do you want children for anyway?' Since that fated day my partner has 'decided' that he didn't want children anyway, doesn't even like them, etc. and just wants us to have a happy life together doing the things we enjoy, despite him feeling upset because 'it would be nice to have the choice'. I, on the other hand, cannot stop my feelings and urges, I can't stop wanting a child even though I know it won't happen. My partner will not consider AID, adoption or fostering, he is simply now a 'closed book'. I love my partner and will not leave him as has been suggested by some 'helpful friends' to 'find a man who can give me a child'. Apart from our situation we get on well and are good friends as well as lovers. But bearing the pain is not easy especially as my partner has become very hardened to my 'baby thing'. I really do believe that most men cannot perceive the yearning a woman has for wanting to have children. I have been told to 'just forget all about that' and that I 'will feel better when I have my change'. *Honestly!!* I have been going through many weird emotions lately and I do not like the bitter person that I am becoming. I seem to cope with friends' existing children and have even taken them out on treats and so on with no problem at all. But what I cannot cope with is my partner's brother's baby and his pregnant sister (my partner is one of three, I am one of two and my brother has been infertile from birth, so no hope of grandchildren at all for my parents let alone myself!)

The main problem is that I feel that I cannot communicate with these people. I do not want any involvement with their children. I do not want to be at their family gatherings, christenings and so on. I feel isolated, peripheral, an outsider. I seem to have nothing to say to them and they have nothing to say to me, we have nothing in common with them, I feel that we are the odd ones out. To make things worse people have noticed that I look miserable and have become introverted in these situations despite my resolve each time to try to be jovial and put on a face. I am currently dreading Christmas even though it is months away. We went away on our own last year but my partner wants to spend time with his family this year so there is no escape. I sometimes wonder why life has to be like this when unwanted newborn babies are found discarded in rubbish crushers. It just isn't fair. I am having difficulty in coping with people's innocent enquiries – 'Isn't it about time . . .?', 'When are you two . . .?', 'Do you want children?', 'Are you planning . . .?', and the stupid assumptions and comments 'You're a career person', (Oh, am I? Thanks for telling me that.) The latest 'gems' include 'You can't go to your grave without having a sprog' (said by a male friend to us both when we both sat silent after being asked when we were going to have a baby etc . . .) A classic was: 'If you want to keep your sanity, don't have children.' (If you want to keep your sanity don't suffer the pain of childlessness or infertility – ignorant idiot!)

Then of course I could always choose to confide in a few trusted people. So far I have been rewarded with my trust being betrayed and our private matters being blabbed to others. Additionally 'understanding' friends will listen as you open your heart, cry, sob and generally fall apart, and will 'help' by saying things like: 'Children aren't everything, you know, but I wouldn't be without mine!' (How very helpful, I'm so glad I told you. I feel so much better about my bereavement now – thanks!?!)

People without partners have problems, too – and they will have no one as close to share their grief with. They will get little sympathy at all, even from infertile couples. And the older woman may well find that her problem is not perceived with much sympathy, either, often subjected to long harangues about how she's near the menopause anyway, and how tiring she'd find it all. And all this delivered, usually, as if these things had never crossed her mind in the first place.

Then there are the mums who already have children, but can't have more for some reason or another – secondary subfertility – who are met by the comforting comment 'Be thankful for the children you've got!' This, despite the fact that mothers with children already may suffer even more. They know what it's like. They have more of a reality to mourn than those who have never had any at all. The following letter is from a woman who has a child already:

Infertility is a difficult subject to discuss at any time, but there is a certain understanding for those who have never had children. When I tell people (rarely) that I am infertile, they cannot understand, as I already have one child. When I explain the circumstances and how desperate I am for another child, the usual reply is: 'At least you have a child, you should be thankful for that.' This gives me tremendous feelings of guilt for wanting another one, when some couples have none. But the overwhelming maternal urges are the same for those with secondary infertility as are the mentions, the desperation, the feelings of failure hard to bear. The lack of understanding makes the situation harder to cope with. You cannot switch off the biological feelings of wanting a child just because you have had one.

'The worst thing about subfertility,' says Jennifer Hunt, 'is that you can often never really get on with grieving until you reach the menopause. The grief is always anticipatory. There always seems to be hope. Until the hopes have finally come to an end, until the thing is finite, it is so hard to grieve.' Which brings us to a new stage altogether: when do you stop trying? When you get pregnant? When you've had X number of tests? When the money runs out? And what do you do then?

8
What next?

It used to be a lot easier to call a halt to fertility treatment. After a certain point, there simply wasn't any more to be had. Then you somehow rearranged your life completely or you simply left the whole thing to chance. But there was something to be said for the power being removed entirely from your hands. You knew you had done your best, you could have done no more and that was it.

These days it could take up to a year simply to get the tests completed. Unless there are very simple and clear results, this could be followed by years and years of treatment.

As long as the money didn't run out, you could go on having IVF attempts for ever. (In the UK a halt would be called around the age of the menopause, but then there is always Italy to run to if you are hell-bent on becoming a grey-haired mother – not to be recommended, however, for obvious reasons, not least that the child would almost certainly suffer.) Some couples find that they are just starting to live with the idea of being subfertile or infertile when some new treatment springs into the arena, and all their hopes are raised over again, along with all the anxieties.

You could try AID, again and again, if it were appropriate; you could try having someone else's egg implanted in you, if you have no ovaries; you could employ a surrogate mother to have your own baby for you, if you have no womb – there is almost no end to the possibilities. You could even, theoretically, put another couple's embryo into another woman's body and then collect it nine months later. The latest dangerously futuristic idea is to collect eggs from aborted foetuses to use for infertile mothers, meaning that the baby that was subsequently born had a natural mother who never actually existed.

The emotional and ethical permutations of parenting offered by new techniques present a minefield for the subfertile would-be parent, offering a weird and bizarre supermarket of choices. Sometimes it almost seems as if there is too much on offer – none of it ideal, of course, but all better than no child at all. How can a couple decide what to do?

Some couples have been known to get it into their heads that somewhere their baby is waiting to be born and that it is up to them to provide the means to make it a reality. If you subconsciously harbour such a misguided but completely understandable idea, stopping treatment is extremely hard, for it may seem as if you are actually denying a mythical child, your child, the chance of life. Scrimping and saving to put yourselves through treatment after treatment may sometimes almost become a substitute for parenting. Just as some parents conscientiously care for their baby from the moment of conception by taking care of their health, subfertile parents may, by trying and trying, in a sense, be parenting even before conception at some level. If this is the trap you have found yourselves in, it may be worth bringing this feeling more out into the open, and wondering what kind of 'parents' you are.

Good parents always consider their child. And if the child is seen to be the primary person to be considered before making decisions about new treatments, then you are already on the road to parenthood, we believe, even if you decide to walk out of the clinic without buying anything. If the technique you choose is one that will mean that the child will suffer unnecessarily in the future, what kind of mum and dad will you be? You will not have been good parents; you will have been a selfish couple, only having a child to satisfy your own needs, not because your aim has been to give your child everything you possibly can.

A child must be able to understand its origins, and you must be able to explain those origins to your child with a completely clear conscience. A child conceived by any technique involving the sperm or egg of people other than its parents, surely has a right to be told about it. This parallels the way that openness is now increasingly being encouraged in cases of adopted children.

However, even bearing this in mind, it is entirely up to you when to call a halt to treatment. But, with a few exceptions, most couples find that after long periods of trying, their hopes may well simply fade. After a fifth failed attempt at IVF, you may both wonder if it is worth putting yourselves through the agony of another disappointment. Doctors may do their best not to influence your choice of how to proceed in any way, but they will inevitably give you clues simply by the tone of their voices and their body language. You will start to realize whether you are a good bet or not. Gradually, you may drop out of treatment programmes and become resigned to being child-less. Alternatively, of course, you might become pregnant.

You may wonder why a book on subfertility should have anything to say on the subject of actual pregnancy, but it is worth mentioning because the pregnancies of the subfertile are sometimes very different from the pregnancies of those who conceive easily. Because of almost certain past disappointments, a pregnancy will not be taken for granted in any way. A couple will take no chances at all. Healthy eating, no alcohol, rest, no digging, or flying . . . the subfertile mother takes much greater care of herself and is often far more anxious than most other mums, who, if it is their first child, are anxious enough anyway. Amazingly, it has been known, in rare cases, for mothers who have had lengthy fertility treatment to have abortions once they become pregnant. Their anxiety has been so great that they cannot stand the terror of actually having a child at last. If you are pregnant and this thought has crossed your mind, don't worry. It is not uncommon, though it is quite uncommon to actually do anything about it.

Subfertile women who become pregnant are terrified of having miscarriages or stillbirths – and even when the baby is born their anxiety doesn't stop there. They may worry about cot-deaths, so at night keep checking whether or not the baby is breathing, and they may find it very difficult to leave the baby even for an hour or so with a grandmother or relation: 'Their anxiety is sky high, and with good reason,' says Jennifer Hunt, 'and if you've fought and battled for this baby, you often deny yourself the right to feel as cheesed off as any other mum when the baby has feeding problems or cries for nights on end. You sometimes don't see your baby quite as other parents see theirs. They can, naturally, feel angry and irritable with their babies now and again, but mothers who have had fertility problems often feel exceptionally guilty if they feel angry with their baby at all.'

But, let's say that, for whatever reason, whether you have become pregnant or decided to terminate treatment, you have decided to stop trying. What now?

The first thought in everyone's mind is adoption. Certainly it's the first thought in the minds of those 'sympathetic' friends we have heard so much about. 'Why don't you adopt?' they say, blithely, as if it were pretty much the same as having a baby, and very easy to do. It's a bit like saying to an opera singer who has lost his vocal chords; 'Why don't you take up the piano instead?' Sure, it's all music, but the piano is quite a different instrument from the voice, and it's not easy to learn. You may not be any good at the piano anyway. You may not *want* to learn. And lots of couples simply don't want to adopt because a child would only be precious if it were *their* child. Any old person's child simply isn't the same.

But, having said all this, what if you *do* want to adopt? Unfortunately, your chances are very slim. 'If you are white and have set your heart on adopting a healthy white baby you should be prepared for a long wait and you should accept that you may eventually be disappointed as very few such children need adoption', says the British Agencies for Adoption and Fostering (BAAF) – see page 145 for the address.

In 1991, although 7171 children were adopted, nearly 3 in every 5 were of school age and only 1 in 8 was under one year old; only 895 babies were adopted.

If you felt able to take on a 'special needs' child – that is, one who is either mentally or physically handicapped or who has been through such a difficult time with their parents and suffered such abuse that its behaviour needs constant attention – you might be lucky. Even so, as BAAF points out, special needs children 'have often been abused, or have behavioural patterns to test new parents to the limit'. An affectionate eight-year-old in a wheelchair subject to screaming fits, say, is not quite the same as a tiny baby wrapped in a pink blanket.

Even if you are lucky enough to find a baby, as the trend is for an open rather than secretive attitude to adoption, it means that the child's mother may have the right to be in contact with the child from time to time. If you want to adopt, you have to be over 21 and if you want to adopt jointly with a partner you have to be married, though a single person or one person in an unmarried couple can adopt. Most agencies usually set upper age limits, however, and, of course, some children will specifically benefit from being adopted by a couple with children. Even if you pass all the criteria on paper, you will still have to undergo rigorous testing by a social worker and doctor.

What about adopting from abroad? As other countries are developing their own adoption and fostering services, it's not as easy as it used to be. If you go ahead, you'll have to contact your local social services or social work department, which will be asked to provide, for the Department of Health, a report on your suitability as adopters, and you'll need to contact the Home Office Immigration and Nationality Department for information about procedures. You can find out more about this from the Overseas Adoption Helpline (see page 145 for the number). However, some people are lucky. The following is the story of a couple who hit the adoption jackpot:

We wrote to every adoption agency I could get the address for. Some came back 'gone away', others came back 'lists closed indefinitely'. One came back from Cleveland Social Services saying their list was opening in April and if we were interested someone would call to see us. This happened in August. We were eligible to join, we passed the criteria (married more than three years, under 36 and ceased fertility treatment). We went to a group session in September for 6 weeks and found out what it meant to adopt a baby. It opened our eyes to issues we hadn't considered. Then the home study started which at times was hard but we came through and were approved by a panel the following June. We were now on their list as approved parents, but were warned we might never be matched with a baby and to go away and get on with the rest of your life, which is difficult when you may get the phone call and have a baby in three days.

After waiting a year we decided to have a holiday in the West Indies and move house as we were beginning to think it wouldn't happen. We moved in December of the next year and our social worker came to see us on New Year's Eve to see the new house and so on and have our six-monthly chat. It was awful. Time was getting on, she said there were few babies around and our ages were against us (36 and we might be too successful!) The fact that we had both worked hard for eight years of our marriage and chose to have a nice home was counting against us.

As you can imagine we had a lousy New Year. However, you have to be positive. On January 1 we decided to have another exotic holiday and if nothing had happened by June when we had to go before the panel again as we had been approved for two years and still without a match, we would make enquiries about adopting from Yugoslavia where we had a contact. We never had to make those decisions. On January 19, 1993 my husband received the phone call – we had a ten-week-old baby son. Nothing can prepare you for the whirl of emotions that engulf you – our prayers had been answered. We saw him the next day at his foster mum's and then went out and did a massive shop. He came to live with us on January 23rd and we couldn't quite believe it. Joshua has brought so many people so much joy and happiness. He is worth all we went through. He was in social services' eyes the 'textbook adoption' from getting the phone call to the court date. There were no hitches and he has a lovely story for us to tell him later. His birth mother has written a letter for us to give to him – she loved him and gave him up so he could have a better start. To anyone going through it, don't give up. Our prayers were answered with a gorgeous son who is our pride and joy. He has slept most nights since we got him and has a smile for everyone – Josh, our long-awaited precious baby son.

After adoption, there are only two further options. One is fostering – a very different ball game to adoption. Foster parents look after children only for short periods, and it's only sometimes that the situation is made permanent. There are regular meetings with birth parents.

And the final suggestion is, why not get a dog? It's the sort of suggestion that would meet with a punch on the nose from most infertile people, but it's not one to cast away without considering because an animal can, in a tiny way, mop up some of the maternal and paternal feelings that gnaw so cruelly at the hearts of people who can't have children. The following letter is from a woman who wrote to the *Daily Mail* in response to someone who asked how on earth she could come to terms with her infertility:

> My husband bought me a dog. We took time selecting the breed. It had to be smallish (to hug and cuddle) and have a long coat (to brush, comb and be referred to as hair.) We chose an eight-week-old Cairn Terrier and called her Amy, a human name. A dog any older than that wouldn't have been a baby and for us wouldn't have had the same effect.
>
> She has cards, presents and cakes at birthdays and Christmas, and we never kennel her – if holiday accommodation won't take her then we don't go! Her name is included on all our letters and cards, and we address her as 'our little girl'. In fact, as far as possible, she is treated like a child.

Perhaps, though, you have decided that if you can't have a baby, then you don't want anything. You will just learn to live with the fact of your infertility. This is clearly the rational answer, but it is so easy to say. Some of you may suffer from feelings of real despair, like this woman:

> Once home from hospital, after another failed treatment, my mind was a turmoil of outrage. Few people could say anything to help. In desperation I turned to my sister for support but discovered myself adrift in a different world from hers – she has two children. We seemed unable to communicate and without

blaming her I recognized my isolation. Left alone, I was over-whelmed by my shame. I was unable to look pregnant women in the eyes, not due to any resentment, but because I was not worthy, I felt.

The shock of the possibility of childlessness sent me into a spiral of depression. For months I wept daily. I played mental games with myself; what would I sacrifice for a child? An arm? A leg? The life of a relative? I ticked them all off, knowing that a child was the only thing that would return some meaning to my life. The idea of no children tormented me. Every time I heard of a friend's pregnancy or news of a birth, the yearning felt like a physical pain. I took solace in being bitter and scornful of other, luckier mothers. I accepted that I was now a failed woman. This is what I thought: the female of the species is there to produce the next generation. That is the foundation on which all other successes are built. How can any building stand up without foundation?

Bearing it alone really is too much to expect of yourself. It is best to be as open as possible, and try hard to feel the warmth of people's kind intentions behind the chill of their sometimes crass remarks. One woman says, when people ask if she has children, 'It's not always that easy.' The other person can then pick up the conversation and ask further or move on to other subjects, but it's worth airing the subject because there are more people out there who may sympathize from first-hand experience than you might think, as the following letter shows:

Childlessness is the hardest burden to bear and to confide in others is hard. Since being pregnant we have found that some of our close friends were in the same situation and perhaps if we had all been a bit more truthful and trustful we could have helped and encouraged each other. There is always someone to listen and who knows sincerely the pain and longing in your heart.

Remember, not every woman you see pushing a pram with a new-born baby in it, fell pregnant the first month. That woman could be me! Our baby was born last month, a gift from God!

And the following story is from someone who found that she really could finally come to terms with the situation – something that most people, quite understandably, never do. 'Living with their grief' is about as close as they can get.

After my last, unsuccessful, treatment, in which I got pregnant for six weeks and then miscarried, I had a dream. I was part of some crack military team which travelled to some distant mountain peak (the first to do so). At the end, I was handed a medal with the word 'submission' engraved on it. This triggered, in my waking life, visions of female strength, of endurance through adversity, by submitting to fate. I decided to act on this dream. I hadn't told anyone of my infertility – my own assumption was that if they knew they would see an image of a frightened, pitiful woman surrounded by despair and lost dreams. Then I saw a different picture; a strong woman who had suffered, but emerged confident of herself and courageous enough to try one more time for her chosen goal. What would stop them seeing me like that instead? Since then things have slowly improved. I can now hold a baby in my arms and enjoy the sensation. I can genuinely feel happy when friends discover they are pregnant. The agony is over.

You could try being Buddhist about it all and simply leave things openended, trusting to chance until the menopause. No doubt a bit of you will think that if you publicly give up worrying, then the baby will miraculously appear, like happiness, which is supposed only to come when you are not looking for it. Unfortunately, life works like this rarely. Alternatively, you could try to persuade yourself that you never really wanted a baby in the first place, that you'd be a lousy mother, and thank goodness fate has taken a difficult decision for you. Any strategy that helps you cope is fine, as long as it suits you.

The other day I looked after a friend's eighteen-month-old child and I found that I was not particularly maternal. For instance she had only been gone ten minutes when I had to change his nappy which was pretty soiled! It must have taken me quarter of an hour and one would have died laughing to watch me. Then getting his shoes on . . . His favourite part of the afternoon was banging the table and getting me to do the same. I can't say I found this too much fun so perhaps the 'meant to be!' bit is true.

If you get trapped in your feelings of grief, naturally it's a time to get counselling. If you have been having treatment, it should have been available to you at the hospital, all the way through. If not, you can contact the British Infertility Counselling Association (BICA – their address is on page 145) and they will tell you where you can contact your nearest counsellor. It is probably best to go to one experienced in fertility problems, even though it is very common for people to start off by having counselling for the grief about their infertility and end up linking their unhappiness to all manner of other past events and losses in their lives. Often the unhappiness about infertility is particularly great because the problem has triggered off all kinds of other unhappinesses buried in the past.

Coming to terms with yourself as a person, rather than longing for a baby to put right the unhappiness in your life, is all part not only of healing, but of a maturity that, in the end, we all have to face. The following letter shows how children simply aren't everything:

I was infertile for 12 miserable years. I did nothing with my life expect long for a baby and await the next infertility treatment. Well, I now have two beautiful healthy children of six and eight. But if I knew then what I know now, how different my life would have been.

I am now making up for lost time. At the age of 40 I am going in for my Advanced Driving Test and am also studying for a bronze life-saving exam with the local swimming club. I love my part-time job and spend evenings out with my girlfriends. I just wish someone had sat and told me how to feel fulfilled in my own achievements before. I didn't find fulfilment in my relationship with my husband. Nor did I find fulfilment when I eventually had my two children. I love my family very much. But they did not provide me with this feeling of self-worth and inner confidence I am slowly gaining. The turning point came when I decided what I really wanted to do for myself. I took up aerobics and became a Samaritan. All of a sudden I had something else to think about. I stopped feeling so sorry for myself and began thinking about other problems that people can suffer. The aerobics made me start to feel good about myself for the first time in years. Within 6 months I had my first miscarriage (in all I had 3), but I celebrated the fact that I had managed to conceive after 12 years of treatment. There was no way that I was going to feel negative about a step nearer my precious goal. I could go on. I have found it difficult to put this into words. But I just hope you will let others know how I feel.

And listen to journalist Libby Purves, who, though she now has two children, herself went through a year of trying for a baby: 'It was long enough to decide exactly how far down the medical garden path I wanted to go', she wrote. 'Not far, I reckoned. I well remember the desolate sense of unfairness and the dislike of other women's bumps. But life is there to be lived as it comes; not wasted in making yourself ill and angry. As John Cleese said in *Clockwise*, "It's not the despair – I can stand the despair. It's the hope." '

She argues that motherhood is not everything: 'Human life in the developed world is longer and more varied than it has ever been. Each of us can know more, see more, live longer, create more and do more good than at any time in human history. Active motherhood is a rewarding, absorbing and enriching phase, but still only a phase, like founding a company or heading a school or seeing a big research project through. It does, of course, start a lifelong relationship, but so does having a brother or a sister or a lover or a true best friend . . . We really must stop putting biological motherhood into a special category of glory and privilege; it is only one glittering thread in the tapestry. Sure, a childless woman misses much; but nobody can have everything. Mothers miss a lot, too. They spend the prime of their lives tired, tied and preoccupied.'

Is there anything left, as comfort? I can only quote Dr Viktor E. Frankl, one of the greatest Austrian psychotherapists since Freud and Jung. In his book *Man's Search for Meaning*, he tells of how a man once consulted him, a man who found his second wife sterile after all his other children had died in Auschwitz. He wrote: 'I observed that procreation is not the only meaning of life, for then life in itself would become meaningless, and something which in itself is meaningless cannot be rendered meaningful merely by its perpetuation.' In other words, life has a meaning beyond reproducing oneself. To find this meaning, for those who are suffering the agony of childlessness, means travelling along a rocky and difficult road. But perhaps, through no choice of your own, you may be forced to find another meaning to life, a meaning that, perhaps, is rarely found among those who are preoccupied with bringing up children.

This may sound dreadfully pious. You may well say that you don't want to find any spiritual meaning in life, you just want a baby in your arms, you want to be a parent. But, perhaps you're not, and you can't be. And perhaps you have to find out, as everyone does in the end when their children leave home, that life involves more than simple perpetuation and bringing up children. It is just something the subfertile and infertile have to learn terribly, horribly early.

When one door is closed, no amount of crying and hammering will ever open it, but other doors will open. There is no choice but to pass through them – yes, kicking, screaming, raging, and weeping if you like – but pass through them all the same, and see what you find the other side.

Useful Addresses

Please send a stamped, self-addressed envelope in each case:

Fertility

CHILD
Suite 219
Caledonian House
98 The Centre
Feltham
Middlesex TW13 4BH
Tel: 0181-893 7110

This is a charitable organization that looks into infertility, and helps its members with advice and counselling. Fact sheets are available on many aspects of infertility, and an excellent newsletter is produced four times a year. Their 24-hour telephone service offers support or advice for members with subfertility or infertility problems.

ISSUE (The National Fertility Association Ltd)
509 Aldridge Road
Great Barr
Birmingham B44 8NA
Tel: 0121-344 4414

ISSUE is the largest and oldest independent support group for people with fertility problems, providing help that includes comprehensive literature, fact sheets, medical updates and a quarterly magazine.

The Human Fertilisation and Embryology Authority (HFEA)
Paxton House
30 Artillery Lane
London E1 7LS
Tel: 0171-377 5077

USEFUL ADDRESSES

NEEDS (National Egg and Embryo Donation Society)
Regional IVF Unit
St Mary's Hospital
Whitworth Park
Manchester M13 0JH
Tel: 0161 276 6000

This society exists to raise awareness of the need for egg and embryo donation, as well as providing information concerning the risks and advantages of donation.

COTS (Childlessness Overcome through Surrogacy)
Loandhu Cottage
Gruids Lairg
Sutherland
Scotland IV27 4EF
Tel: 0549 402401 (Helpline and Faxline)

Miscarriage Assocation
c/o Clayton Hospital
Northgate
Wakefield
West Yorkshire WF1 3JS

British Infertility Counselling Association (BICA)
c/o Marilyn Crawshaw
Dakins
Walker Fold Road
Bolton BL1 7PU

Alternative medicine

The Institute for Complementary Medicine
PO Box 194
London SE16 1QZ
Tel: 0171-237 5165

Gives information about complementary practitioners in most areas.

Adoption

Overseas Adoption Helpline
Tel: 0171-226 7666

National Fostercare Association
Leonard House
5–7 Marshalsea Road
London SE1 1EP
Tel: 0171 828 6266

British Agencies for Adoption and Fostering (BAAF)
Skyline House
200 Union Street
London SE1 0OY
Tel: 0171-593 2000

Parent-to-Parent Information on Adoption Service (PPIAS)
The Laurels
Lower Boddington
Near Daventry
Northamptonshire NN11 6YB
Tel: 0327 60295

Donor insemination

D.I. Network
PO Box 265
Sheffield S3 7YX

This is a group started by parents of children conceived by D.I. who have decided to tell their children about their origins and who have come together to support each other and those contemplating D.I. or undergoing treatment.

The network has a list of people who are prepared to talk about their experiences of D.I. and to listen and offer advice and support.

Further Reading

Murphy, Sarah, *Talking About Miscarriage* (Sheldon Press, 1992).

Snowden, R., and Snowden, E. *The Gift of a Child* (Exeter University Press, 1993).

Tan, S. L., and Jacobs, H. S., *Infertility: Your questions answered* (McGraw-Hill Book Co., 1991).

D.I. Network, *My Story* (Infertility Research Trust, 1991). A simple book for parents of D.I. children aged around 4–5 years old. The delightfully illustrated book presents the details in a straightforward and sensitive way, enabling parents to explain how their D.I. children were conceived. Available from:

The Infertility Research Trust
University Department of Obstetrics and Gynaecology
Jessop Hospital for Women
Sheffield S8 0TZ

Index